# THE GREAT PHYSICIAN'S

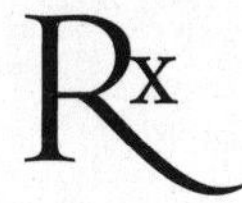

*for*

# WOMEN'S HEALTH

JORDAN AND NICKI RUBIN
with Pancheta Wilson, M.D.

NELSON BOOKS
A Division of Thomas Nelson Publishers
*Since 1798*

www.thomasnelson.com

Every effort has been made to make this book as accurate as possible. The purpose of this book is to educate. It is a review of scientific evidence that is presented for information purposes. No individual should use the information in this book for self-diagnosis, treatment, or justification in accepting or declining any medical therapy for any health problems or diseases. No individual is discouraged from seeking professional medical advice and treatment, and this book is not supplying medical advice. Any application of the information herein is at the reader's own discretion and risk. Therefore, any individual with a specific health problem or who is taking medications must first seek advice from his personal physician or health-care provider before starting a nutrition program. The author and Thomas Nelson Publishers, Inc., shall have neither liability nor responsibility to any person or entity with respect to loss, damage, or injury caused or alleged to be caused directly or indirectly by the information contained in this book. We assume no responsibility for errors, inaccuracies, omissions, or any inconsistency herein.

In view of the complex, individual nature of health and fitness problems, this book, and the ideas, programs, procedures, and suggestions are not intended to replace the advice of trained medical professionals. All matters regarding one's health require medical supervision. A physician should be consulted prior to adopting any program or programs described in this book. The author and publisher disclaim any liability arising directly or indirectly from the use of this book.



Published in Nashville, Tennessee, by Thomas Nelson, Inc.

Nelson Books titles may be purchased in bulk for educational, business, fund-raising, or sales promotional use. For information, please e-mail SpecialMarkets@ThomasNelson.com.



**Library of Congress Cataloging-in-Publication Data**

Rubin, Jordan.
The great physician's Rx for women's health / by Jordan and Nicki Rubin with Pancheta Wilson.
p. cm.
Includes bibliographical references.
ISBN-13: 978-0-7852-1901-9 (hardcover)
ISBN-10: 0-7852-1901-3
ISBN-13: 978-0-7852-8894-7 (IE)
ISBN-10: 0-7852-8894-5
1. Women—Health and hygiene. I. Rubin, Nicki. II. Wilson, Pancheta. III. Title.
RA778.R778 2006
613'.04244—dc22 2006034500

*Printed in the United States of America*

1 2 3 4 5 RRD 10 09 08 07 06

To Grandma Ruth, our mothers Phyllis and Jane, our sisters Jenna and Angela, we pray your lives will be filled with hope, health, and happiness.

# Contents

# Introduction

**From Jordan Rubin:** Not long after the release of the *Great Physician's Rx for Health and Wellness,* I knew without hesitation that I wanted my next book to address the health concerns of women.

I had several reasons for feeling this way. While my previous books have been universally well received by both sexes, women have been *more* receptive to my message regarding what God says about living a long, healthy, and abundant life. I base this observation on the thousands of phone calls and e-mails I've received from females and the long lines of determined women waiting to have a word with me whenever I sign books or speak at churches and conferences, like Women of Faith.

Women, much to my masculine chagrin, are the ones asking the right questions and seeking the right answers. Most guys pay far too little attention to what they eat or how much they exercise until—boom!—they suffer a major health crisis, such as a heart attack.

It's also my steadfast belief that women—who are not only responsible for their own health but frequently for the health of their husbands, children, and often their aging parents—are sick and tired of being sick and tired. They simply want more out of life and have an intuitive sense that there's more to good health than barely getting through a long day of family-related tasks and wifely duties. To them, it's about thriving, not just surviving. Women are beginning to recognize that there has to be a better route to wellness than sitting in a doctor's examination room, engaging in a cursory three-minute dialogue with a harried physician and exiting with a prescription in hand.

Still, the idea of charging ahead and writing a book on women's health all by my lonesome didn't feel like the right thing to do. After all, *I'm a man!* While I consider myself to be a very sensitive guy, even someone as understanding as myself could never think or communicate like a woman. How could I, a red-blooded American male living in a men-are-from-Mars/women-are-from-Venus world, possibly address the areas of wellness pertinent to a woman's health? I was sure that my advice would prompt my female readers to roll their eyes.

But what if I teamed up with a woman who knows *exactly* what I think about living the healthiest life possible? What if I joined forces with a woman who understands my heart, my thoughts, and my passion for good health—a woman who grew up eating the typical all-American diet, but who was exposed to the Bible's health plan and benefited greatly from following the Great Physician's prescription for health and wellness?

The more I thought about it, the more I realized that there is only one person suited for this job: my wife, Nicki, who's an exemplary spouse and loving mom to our two-year-old son, Joshua.

**From Nicki:** When Jordan asked me what I thought about joining him in the *Great Physician's Rx for Women's Health*, I thought, *Hmmm . . . this could be interesting*. Granted, he's quite familiar and even empathetic with the health issues that women face, but the fact that he *isn't* a woman means that he will never fully understand the more sensitive health issues we face, such as hormonal concerns, our "time of the month," infertility, or the first trimester of pregnancy.

Therefore, I believe that I'm the best person to come alongside Jordan because I understand his passion better than anyone else. I've been exposed to and personally benefited from his message on healthy living for about ten years, and I can assure you that he's the real deal.

We are also thrilled to have our contributing coauthor and medical editor, Pancheta Wilson, MD, a family and complementary medicine physician from Coral Springs, Florida, lend to our book her vast experience as a doctor and a godly woman.

Eating healthy and enjoying the benefits of an active lifestyle have been Jordan's passion for more than a decade, and he loves to share his passion with others. His dogged determination to eat a steady diet of whole and natural foods, take the highest-quality supplements, practice advanced hygiene, exercise, reduce toxins in his environment, avoid deadly emotions, and live a life of prayer and purpose stems from his college days, when he got *really* sick.

Following Jordan's freshman year at Florida State University, he was a counselor at a Christian summer camp when he began experiencing "health challenges." As he described in greater detail in *The Great Physician's Rx for Health and Wellness*, Jordan nearly died after months and months of intense pain and suffering. At one point, when he was down to 104 pounds, his doctors recommended an ostomy—the removal of his large intestine and part of his small intestine. I'm sure that sounded like a fate worse than death to a twenty-year-old guy.

After visiting more than seventy doctors and health experts, and trying dozens of conventional treatments and hundreds of exotic "cures" for what supposedly ailed him, Jordan turned to the Bible for answers to his devastating health problems. He shared his discoveries in the *Great Physician's Rx for Health and Wellness*, including his belief that too many people coast through life without realizing that at least 80 percent of their diseases are lifestyle related. Too few Americans understand the significance of what they eat; the quantities they consume; or the effects of a sedentary yet fast-paced, high-stress lifestyle on their health.

Jordan has come up with a concise and simple way to convey his advice for living a healthy life—outlined in what he terms the "Seven Keys to Unlocking Your Health Potential."

The Seven Keys are:

Key #1: Eat to live.

Key #2: Supplement your diet with whole food nutritionals, living nutrients, and superfoods.

Key #3: Practice advanced hygiene.

Key #4: Condition your body with exercise and body therapies.

Key #5: Reduce toxins in your environment.

Key #6: Avoid deadly emotions.

Key #7: Live a life of prayer and purpose.

In the *Great Physician's Rx for Women's Health,* we will be adapting and customizing each of these keys to the unique needs of women. You'll find in this book a lot of great information that you can put to good use right away.

The desire in both of our hearts is contained in an old African proverb: "Educate a man, and you educate an individual. Educate a woman, and you educate a family." As you read through this book, Jordan and I implore you to incorporate these timeless principles and allow the living God to transform your health and your life.

## WOMEN *Are* DIFFERENT THAN MEN

**Jordan:** Before we go farther, we need to set the table regarding the state of women's health in this country. It's a toss-up on whether women are healthier than men, but if women are healthier, it's only by a nose.

*Majority Rules*

In demographic terms, women outnumber men in the U.S. 50.8 to 49.2 percent; in real numbers, that's around 150 million women to 145 million men, according to the latest United States Census statistics.[1]

**Nicki:** I tend to believe that it's too difficult to say whether men are healthier than women, or vice versa—you're comparing apples to oranges. Maybe when boys are younger, they are more athletically minded than girls and participate in more calorie-burning activities, which makes them appear healthier. But when girls get older, they become very concerned about their appearance, which prompts them to pay attention to their weight, what they eat, and how much they exercise. So it's difficult to determine which sex is healthier. In my own experience as a new mother, I've discovered that something has to give when the demands of motherhood take precedence. A mom will overlook her own health before neglecting her children's care.

**Jordan:** Good point. I began the introduction of my book *The Maker's Diet* by writing about the hypothetical Average Jane: a married mother, age thirty-seven, who wore size 16 pants and thirty extra pounds, mostly on her hips and thighs. "Jane" lacked energy and didn't feel particularly healthy, but her husband was even more overweight and out of shape than she. Her flabby children were afflicted with a host of juvenile maladies, including obesity, attention deficit hyperactivity disorder, and allergies, yet Jane's idea of a nutritious sack lunch for them was a slice of honey-glazed ham slapped on "fortified" Wonder bread, a handful of reduced-fat Oreos tucked inside a resealable plastic bag, and a box of Capri Sun with 10 percent fruit juice. Jane's father had died of a massive heart attack before his time, and her mother was battling painful arthritis and the beginnings of dementia.

This Average Jane, in the prime of her life, was responsible not only for raising demanding children, dependent on her for both emotional nurturing and nutritional sustenance, but also for looking after her husband, her aging parents, and her in-laws. I'm sure that what I am describing is not new to you. The bulk of both child rearing and caring for the immediate and extended family have fallen squarely on the shoulders of women since the beginning of time, although there are certainly exceptions.

It seems that the Lord God almighty, in His infinite wisdom, created women to be more nurturing and relational than men. This has a stabilizing effect on marriages, and balances home life. Though the discussion of God's intent for men and women to have distinct but equally important roles in society is beyond the scope of this book, we must recognize that the Lord created the different sexes to complement and complete each other. While men typically act more aggressively and have the single-minded drive to accomplish tasks, women tend to be more supportive. Whereas women value love, communication, beauty, and relationships, a man's sense of self is often defined by his ability to achieve results.

When I was growing up in the '70s and '80s, feminists argued that there were no essential differences between the sexes, and the patriarchal and matriarchal roles observed in society were due to conditioning. I remember neighbor kids whose parents were careful not to let their boys go wild with "Cowboys and Indians," or their girls to play house with their Barbie dolls. But as social scientists unearthed evidence dispelling the idea that men and women were essentially the same underneath the obvious physical differences, the social pendulum began swinging the other way. These days, the prevailing conventional wisdom is that, well, women are different from men. And just as males and females have significant biological and physiological differences, there are also noteworthy distinctions in the area of health.

Women possess only two-thirds of the overall physical strength of men, but a woman's abdominal muscles contain just as much strength as a male's. This was part of God's design for women because a pregnant woman needs strong abdominal muscles for childbirth. Additionally, according to the Mayo Clinic:

- women, on average, have 11 percent more body fat and 8 percent less muscle mass than men;
- men tend to be faster than women during aerobic events due to their great muscle strength and the mechanical advantage of longer arms and legs;
- women, on the other hand, tend to have greater endurance, partly due to reliance on fat metabolism, during long events;
- though women scream "Ouch!" in pain before men do, they tolerate the pain better than men do.[2]

Dr. James Dobson noted some important differences between men and women in his book *Love for a Lifetime.* For instance, women have larger stomachs, kidneys, livers, and appendixes. Their thyroid glands are also generally larger and more active, usually enlarging during both menstruation and pregnancy. This makes them more prone to developing goiters and more vulnerable in cold weather. It is also associated with smooth skin and a relatively hairless body. A woman's blood contains 20 percent fewer red blood cells than a male's, which means her blood contains more water. Since blood carries oxygen to the body's cells, fewer red blood cells means less oxygen is made available: women tire more easily. Finally, a woman's heart beats more rapidly (eighty beats per minute versus seventy-two for men), but she has much less tendency to develop high blood pressure.[3]

So are women healthier than men? Well, women do live longer—5.3 years, according to the Centers for Disease Control and Prevention, but the "gender gap" between male and female life expectancy has been narrowing since the peak gap of 7.8 years was recorded in 1979.[4] The reason for the gap remains a mystery.

**Nicki:** I wonder if the gap is narrowing because of the millions of career-minded women who entered the workforce in the 1970s and '80s. Since men have a shorter lifespan presumably because they work at high-pressure jobs and stress themselves out of a few years, I would think that being a mom *and* holding down a full-time job outside the home could also cut off some years.

**Jordan:** You could be right, but Dr. Eugenia Eng told students at the University of North Carolina: "Women are sicker; men die quicker."[5] I guess women are like Timex watches: they take a licking but keep on ticking. Yet my research shows that more women than men die from the nation's number-one killer—cardiovascular disease—each year. If you're keeping score, women have a 53 to 47 percent edge. According to the American Heart Association, the number of deaths from heart disease among females has exceeded those of males since 1984.[6]

Furthermore, one in three women has some form of cardiovascular disease, yet only 13 percent of women are aware that heart disease is a major threat to their lives.[7] They think that only men keel over, clutching their chests as everything fades to black during a fatal heart attack. The fact is, women account for nearly half of all deaths from heart attack.[8]

When it comes to the second leading cause of death—cancer—a slightly higher percentage of men than women go to the grave each year. The most common form of cancer deaths among women is lung cancer, not breast cancer, as is often believed. Nearly twice the number of women perish annually from lung cancer as compared to breast cancer (74,000 to 40,000), yet we do not see pink ribbons or 10K walks for lung cancer.[9] And what gets me is that no one is talking about how 60 percent of all cancers in women can be linked to dietary and lifestyle factors.[10]

In addition, women are twice as likely as men to die from both stroke and Alzheimer's disease, a progressive, degenerative brain disease that starts as slight memory loss and degenerates into irreversible mental impairment.[11] And though diabetes—which is the leading cause of blindness, kidney failure, limb amputations, and heart disease—preys slightly more on men than women, 9 percent of women over the age of twenty have diabetes, and one-third of them don't even know it, according to the American Diabetes Association.[12]

*Nag Him to Good Health*
*by Jordan Rubin*

> *A nagging wife is as annoying as the constant dripping on a rainy day.*
> Proverbs 27:15 (NLT)

King Solomon wrote this 3,000 years ago, but he probably didn't know back then that nagging may add years to a person's life.

If you're thinking, *Huh?*, let me explain. While nagging can be irritating, some friendly, good-natured badgering from wife to husband can help men live longer and enjoy better health. That's the thesis of a book, *The Case for Marriage,* written by University of Chicago researcher Linda Waite, and Maggie Gallagher, president of the Institute for Marriage and Public Policy.

"Marriage provides individuals—and especially men—with someone who monitors their health and health-related behaviors and who encourages self-regulation," said Linda Waite, adding that married men can benefit from "someone who nags them."[13]

Wives have a way of getting husbands to give up what we call "stupid bachelor tricks," such as driving fast, drinking in bars, and getting into fights. They can, at the same time, participate in improving their husband's health by cooking healthier meals (*anything* is healthier than what passes for many young bachelors' diets). They can also encourage their men to get regular sleep, to slap sunscreen on their noses, and to visit their doctors for their annual prostate exams. (Thanks a lot, Sweetie!)

So the next time you find yourself nagging—uh—*encouraging* your husband to lay off the Pringles and clam dip before dinner, remember the potential long-term health benefits from your pestering.

Finally, twice as many women suffer from symptoms of irritable bowel syndrome (IBS)—recurring constipation, abdominal pain, digestive discomfort, and bloating—than men. Chronic constipation in women contributes to the development of hemorrhoids, diverticulosis, and polyp formation.

Though these are sobering statistics, I know that women by nature are more proactive about their health than men. They are more likely to visit a doctor, consult with a pharmacist, read a diet book, and take nutritional supplements such as vitamins and minerals. Men, on the other hand, are more likely to "tough it out" when they experience medical symptoms, according to an ACNielsen research study.[14] And though men use the Internet more frequently than women, women are more likely to search the Web for answers to their health questions or concerns.[15]

Women—and realize that I'm generalizing here and not trying to sound sexist—set the tone for nearly all aspects of good health in the home: they are usually the ones doing the grocery shopping, preparing the meals, and doing most of the housecleaning. If they're mothers, they're making sure everyone takes their vitamins, bathing the younger ones, insisting on good hygiene practices, getting kids to bed on time, and setting the emotional thermostat in the home. And in many households these days, those things happen after a long day at work.

No wonder women report feeling tired all the time. As I see how well Nicki handles everything around our home, I marvel at how far she has come in terms of living a healthy lifestyle because when we were dating, I had my doubts.

**Nicki:** I'll never forget some of our conversations when we were dating. Jordan asked me a lot of general questions, including, "Do you think you're healthy?"

I was in my mid-twenties at the time, traveling through life at my physical peak. I actually looked him in the eye and said, "I'm one of the healthiest people I know."

He didn't smirk, and he didn't give me one of those know-it-all looks. (That would come later.) Instead, he cleared his throat and respectfully asked me, "Why do you say that?"

"Because I haven't had any soda since I was seventeen, and I don't eat fast food," I declared. In my mind, those two actions qualified me as one of the healthiest people I knew. I thought I was doing pretty well for someone who grew up in a three-stoplight town called Paintsville, Kentucky, population 5,300, two hours east of Lexington and close to the West Virginia border.

One of our family rules was that we always sat down for dinner together. Mom did most of the cooking, so her mantra was, *It has to be quick and easy.* Occasionally she served those frozen turkey-and-gravy meals that you heat up in the oven, but most of the time it was hot dogs and hamburgers, spaghetti, or my all-time, least-favorite meal: salmon cakes, pinto beans, and cornbread.

Weekends were special because Mom made a big breakfast of biscuits and gravy (made with bacon fat, white flour, and milk), scrambled eggs, and bacon. Saturday nights were often reserved for *homemade* pizza layered with lots of pepperoni and cheese. My favorite meal of the week was Sunday dinner, when Mom really made a special meal. She would cut up a chicken and fry it in Wesson oil (which was better than the Crisco she used previously) until it was golden brown. Then she would prepare scalloped potatoes from a box and our favorite vegetable dish—broccoli casserole, which included crumbled Ritz crackers, a fistful of margarine, and a block of Velveeta cheese.

Mom filled our cupboards with various convenience foods and drinks, and I was in charge of making the tea in our house. In Kentucky, the only kind of tea is *sweet* tea. After brewing a gallon of Lipton tea, I would dump an entire cup of white sugar into the container. I began drinking sweet tea in the sixth grade, and it became my drink of choice.

As far as I knew, I ate and drank what everyone else in America ate and drank, but thankfully I had a pretty fast metabolism as I hit the teen years. I started becoming more health conscious in high school after my science teacher suggested an experiment. "I want you to drop a nail into a glass of Coke," he said at the beginning of class one day, "and observe the acidic reaction." Now, the nail didn't dissolve over the next few days—that's an old wives' tale—but the red rust and gritty corrosion on the galvanized nail blew me away. "That's what happens to your stomach," my teacher declared at the end of the experiment.

I was convinced. From that day forward, I decided to shun soft drinks, but I picked up a jag for sweet, flavored coffees while studying for an accounting degree at Morehead State College in Morehead, Kentucky. Mocha and French vanilla became my favorites. And I still had a thing for sweet tea.

After I graduated from college and was out on my own for a few years, I applied for a position with a Big 5 accounting firm, Arthur Andersen, which had a branch office situated in West Palm Beach along Florida's Treasure Coast. The thought of never shoveling snow and maintaining a year-round tan sounded great, so I packed my Honda Prelude and moved to West Palm Beach without knowing a soul.

I checked into a local hotel to get my bearings, where a friendly bellman suggested that I attend Christ Fellowship Church in nearby Palm Beach Gardens. It didn't take long for a friendly guy to invite me to attend their singles' group, called Souled Out Singles, which met on Monday nights.

When I first walked in that Monday evening, I noticed several guys and gals standing around a tall, handsome guy with black hair.

"You should have been here last week," a young man said to me. "Jordan shared his testimony about how he nearly died from this awful illness, and how God healed him."

And that's how I was introduced to Jordan Rubin.

"Hey, Jordan, show Nicki that photo," said his acquaintance.

Jordan opened his Bible and flashed a snapshot taken of him a couple of years earlier. I barely recognized the ghastly figure with dark legs that looked like skin over bone and a rib cage exposed from the loss of so much weight.

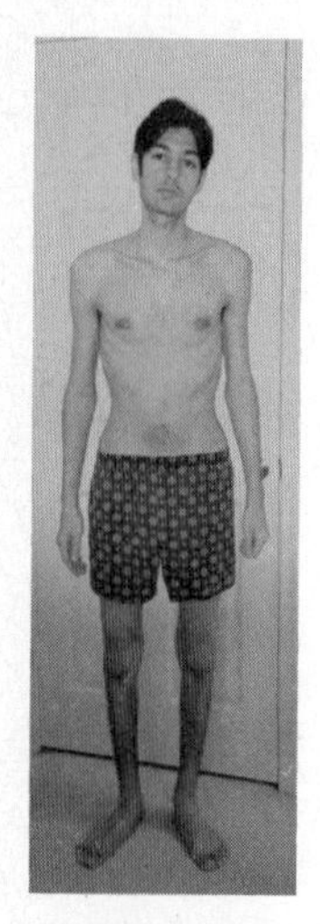

BEFORE

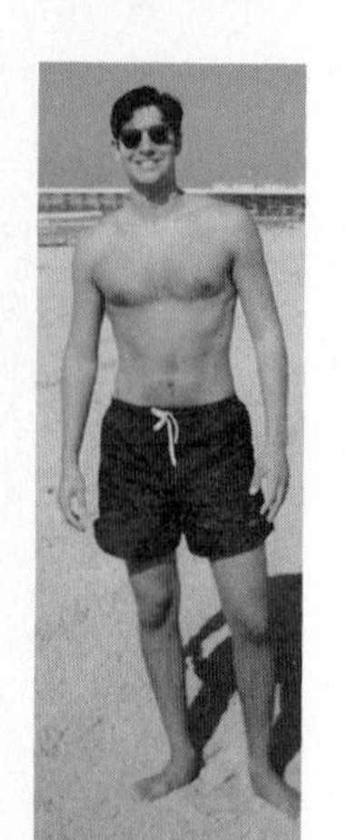

AFTER

"That can't be you!" I said in disbelief.

"That was me," he replied with a shy smile.

I could barely see the resemblance between the fit, tanned, energetic guy standing in front of me and the walking skeleton posing in front of a white closet door.

That evening, we became casual friends in the Souled Out Singles group. Over the next few weeks, I ran into Jordan several times. We became close friends, and after six months, we started dating. I noticed that he liked to talk about two things: the Bible and health. Those were his two big passions, along with a little baseball and music thrown in.

"So, do you consider yourself a healthy person?" he asked me one night while we were on a date.

Well, I *looked* like a healthy person, so I answered him quite confidently. I thought he might actually be impressed when I told him that I hadn't had a soda in ten years, didn't eat fast food, drank only fat-free milk, ate lots of fruit and veggies, and rarely had dessert.

From the expression on Jordan's face, I could tell that he wasn't impressed.

That's when I decided I didn't dare disclose that I sometimes drank a gallon of sweet tea a day, occasionally devoured a large bag of strawberry-flavored Twizzlers in one sitting, or consumed chips and salsa like they were one of the four food groups.

That evening Jordan was content to let me talk because he knew that I was open to his advice. Since he also thought this relationship was leading to the altar, he didn't want to overwhelm me with his views on what constituted a healthy lifestyle. So he kept everything low-key, and I'm sure it helped that I was obviously interested in living a healthy life.

And after six months of friendship, a year of dating, and a seven-month engagement, I became Mrs. Jordan Rubin. But a thought came to me as I departed Christ Fellowship under a rain of soap bubbles and "best wishes" that afternoon: *Who will do the grocery shopping after our honeymoon?* Despite my growing interest in health, I was not as radical as Jordan when it came to what I ate.

As it turned out, the adjustment would be *pretty* radical . . .

# Key #1

## *Eat to Live*

**Nicki:** Growing up, Mom tried to teach me her favorite time-tested recipes, but for some reason, the basics of Southern cuisine escaped me. My cooking experience was limited to frying Steak-ums in a saucepan, heating spuds in a microwave, and making sweet tea by the gallon.

In college, I didn't have to cook because I could rely on dorm food, Hot Pockets, or fast food for sustenance. But when I got out on my own and realized that I couldn't afford two restaurant meals a day, I told myself that I had better expand my cooking abilities, or I would be destined to relive each dinner like in *Groundhog Day.* Back then I couldn't summon the culinary skills necessary even to fry drumsticks. Boiling water was about the range of my kitchen talent.

Fortunately for me, my roommates were often content to cook for the both of us from the time I left college until the day I exchanged marriage vows with Jordan. Unfortunately for my newlywed husband, he married someone with limited cooking skills—and an even more limited desire to cook.

I'm sure that Jordan, following our honeymoon, was in a state of shock when he discovered my appalling lack of aptitude in the kitchen. But eating out every night would have blown a hole in our finances, so that wasn't a viable option. Since Jordan was into health foods and I wasn't, we decided that he would shop at a local health food store for what he liked to eat, and I would buy my favorite foods at a supermarket. This was fine with me because I knew how important it was to Jordan to eat natural and organic foods; I had gotten that message loud and clear during our courting days.

To illustrate how silly the food détente became, he carried home plastic sacks filled with free-range chicken, organic vegetables, and snacks such as organic blueberries. Meanwhile, I filled my shopping cart with Tyson chicken and "regular" fruits and veggies. My snacks were convenience foods like tortilla chips and bottled salsa. Jordan purchased organic Gala apples; I preferred shiny (and waxy) Red Delicious apples from Publix because they were prettier to my eye.

I know—pretty ridiculous, but I was tenaciously hanging on to the foods I had grown up with. But Jordan was very smart: he knew better than to compel me to eat his way, so he started slowly. Once, after dinner, he offered me a Pamela's Espresso Chocolate Chunk Cookie, which was a wheat-free organic treat. Now that pleased my sweet tooth! I probably finished the box that night. On another occasion, I sampled his baked French fries from Cascadian Farm, dipped in organic ketchup. *Way* tastier than fast-food fries cooked in heavy grease!

Over the next few weeks, I sampled more of the organic fruits, veggies, and natural foods that my husband had purchased—and they tasted better and felt "cleaner" as they made their way through my system. Each bite produced a starburst of flavors. I began to think, *Maybe there's something to eating this healthy stuff.*

Sometime toward the end of our first year of marriage, I made a conscious, deliberate switch: whatever Jordan ate, I ate. But I still wasn't handy in the kitchen. Dinner at our place was like trolling the buffet table at a Super Bowl party: one night we'd eat organic chips and salsa; the next night I would set out organic cheese and blanched almonds. To break up the monotony, I would dice up pineapple, melons, and strawberries. Bottom line, I didn't feel confident enough to tackle a hot meal from scratch.

I could tell that Jordan, who was no Iron Chef in the kitchen either, was becoming exasperated. He was busy launching a health and wellness company that demanded insane hours, but my schedule with the Arthur Andersen accounting firm was even *more* intense. By the time I got home from my numbing, hour-long commute, I was shot from the long day and cranky from hunger. Popping a pair of Amy's organic pizzas into the oven summoned all of my remaining energy.

But after Jordan casually mentioned one night that we sure seemed to be eating a lot of organic pizza, I decided to give cooking a try. Even *I* could dice up chicken breasts and brown them in a frying pan. When I was done, I would ladle them atop a simple salad. Or I would cook fresh fish or meat in a saucepan, along with some organic vegetables. I discovered that garlic and butter could make *anything* taste good.

I added eggs to my repertoire because Jordan shared with me that eggs were nutritional powerhouses, nutrient-dense food that packed six grams of protein—*plus* vitamins B-12, E, and D, lutein, riboflavin, calcium, zinc, iron, and essential fatty acids—into a mere seventy-five calories. That was news to me. All I had ever heard was that eggs were high in cholesterol and could clog up your arteries.

Jordan suggested that I scramble the eggs in extra-virgin coconut oil—instead of margarine or vegetable oil—because coconut oil is high in healthy fats called medium-chain fatty acids. I began scrambling several eggs in extra-virgin coconut oil and found that scrambled eggs mixed with some goat's feta cheese made an excellent breakfast or dinner.

I had heard it said that if you can read, you can cook, so I tackled my first homemade soup by following a recipe I found in an excellent cookbook, *Nourishing Traditions.* Dice an onion? I could do that. Peel and chop carrots and celery? No problem. Measure out water and add organic chicken? Easy as pie. Chicken soup became a staple early in our marriage.

**Jordan:** After seven years together, you wouldn't recognize Nicki in the kitchen today. She could give Rachael Ray of the Food Network a run for her money. Nicki probably cooks from scratch four or five nights a week. And I like rolling up my sleeves and cooking for the family as well. Recently I made Thai Coconut Chicken Soup, a phenomenal organic salad with salmon, avocado, and fresh herbs and spices—all topped off with coconut chocolate mouse pudding. When I can't pitch in, I'm happy to report that Nicki is way beyond making reservations for dinner. When I have ministry partners in town, I'd rather invite them to our house to feast on Nicki's spinach-and-goat-cheese lasagna, made with ground buffalo meat, than to take a chance at finding something decent to eat in a restaurant.

These days Nicki loves to experiment with recipes and fashion meals that are tastier and even healthier. She contributed two dozen recipes to the *Great Physician's Rx for Health and Wellness* as well.

**Nicki:** We like to eat under our own roof because we enjoy eating fresh, homemade meals. Sure, I enjoy dining at nice restaurants, but I like to reserve eating out for special occasions. Jordan and I are content to eat at our dining room table because we know that our meal is going to be healthier and better tasting than what we could find in restaurants. One of my favorites recipes is a meat loaf made from grass-fed beef, bison, or venison. I adorn this delicious dish with real mashed potatoes made with organic heavy whipping cream and real butter. My way of thinking in the kitchen has changed to this: if I'm going to go to the trouble to cook a meal from scratch, then I want to use the best ingredients possible. Then the meal not only tastes better, but it's much better for you. We pretty much eat all organic all the time: meat and vegetables, eggs and fruit, cheese and nuts. And anything with mushrooms is great for me.

**Jordan:** Our philosophy behind good food is based on the first key to unlocking your health potential, which is "Eat to live." This principle involves choosing something that will be better for your body in the long term rather than a quick fix to squelch cravings. The apostle Paul described the attitude we should have about food and eating in 1 Corinthians 6:13 (TLB), with a small addition by me: "For instance, take the matter of eating. God has given us an appetite for food and stomachs to digest it. But that doesn't mean we should eat more than we need. Don't think of eating as [overly] important, because some day God will do away with both stomachs and food."

Sadly, too many people "live to eat"—they indulge their palates with deep-fried, high-calorie, high-sodium, high-sugar, and high-fat foods that are also high in taste—or so they believe. Many are unaware that their taste buds have been manipulated by fast-food restaurants and food conglomerates that slap breaded coatings on chicken, sweeten meats with "secret sauces," and cover everything else with bacon and melted cheese.

Fast food is the antithesis of eating to live, but meals-on-the-go are a popular option for harried women (some who've worked outside the home all day) trying to get their kids fed after a long day of carpooling, piano lessons, and soccer games.

Moms, you know the scenario: It's 6 p.m., and you've just picked up your last child from team practice. You're tired, it's getting dark, the kids are cranky and hungry, and you don't have anything in the refrigerator. So you follow the path of least resistance and turn into a McDonald's drive-thru, where you're handed a sack of Happy Meals for the kids and a Bacon Ranch Salad with crispy chicken for you—including a packet of high-fat creamy buttermilk dressing. (And when you're single, it hardly seems worth it to fix a healthy and nutritious meal for just one person.)

What I've described is commonplace since 70 million fast-food meals are served daily across the fruited plain, from behemoth chains like Mickey D's to upstarts like Chipotle. Fast-food restaurants are as abundant as street lamps and found on every main boulevard and commercial thoroughfare in America.

The problem with fast food—or any sort of meal-on-the-go, like TV dinners, turkey potpies, or chicken nuggets—is that you and your family are eating processed foods that God definitely did not create and in a form not healthy for your body. Anytime your dinner is assembled by teens in paper hats or line workers in hair nets, you can be sure you're eating foods that have been adulterated with sugars, salt, chemically charged additives, and unhealthy preservatives that make them cheaper to mass-produce—and more appealing to your tainted taste buds.

That will need to change. The idea behind Key #1 is to eat what God created for food, and in a form healthy for the body. I'm convinced that a diet based on whole and natural foods is the bull's-eye of eating to live. And, as Nicki discovered, healthy food can and does taste great.

## STOCKING UP

So, what kinds of foods should be finding their way to your cupboard and refrigerator? Well, a few examples are whole grains like wheat and barley; nuts and seeds; healthy dairy product like yogurt, cheese, and butter; fish and fowl; fruits and veggies such as berries, tomatoes, and avocados; and healthy red meats like beef, lamb, venison, and bison. These foods, which come as close to nature as possible, will nourish your body, sustain energy throughout the long day, and give you the best chance to live the healthiest life possible. Whole and natural foods are especially important for young bodies because bones, muscle, and sinew only grow to maturation once. That's why I'm a proponent of natural foods grown organically or raised sustainably, because God created these foods in a form healthy for the body.

### *Shopping for Organic Food*
*by Nicki Rubin*

Shopping in health food stores, like Whole Foods Market or Wild Oats, is becoming more and more popular as women discover the benefits of natural and organic versus conventional foods. Nearly two-thirds of U.S. consumers purchased organic foods and beverages in 2005, up from about half in 2004, according to *Consumer Reports*. During the past decade, sales of organic foods have grown 20 percent or more annually.[1]

No longer do you have to shop in out-of-the-way stores for organic foods. Major grocery chains like Safeway, Vons, Kroger, Fred Meyer, Ralphs, Publix, Winn-Dixie, and Albertsons are dedicating entire aisles to organic foods. Costco has added organic eggs, milk, fruit and vegetables, and wild-caught salmon and tuna. Even Wal-Mart, the world's biggest retailer, is responding to market forces. In 2006, Wal-Mart doubled its organic offerings and developed a plan to encourage fisheries to adopt Marine Stewardship Council practices so that it could sell more wild-caught fish.[2] Sam's Club, owned by Wal-Mart, also began offering "sensational low prices" on organic foods.

Wal-Mart's entry into the organic-food market could change the shopping landscape in years to come, but for now, many moms balk at the cost of going organic. Organic fruits, vegetables, meats, and eggs are more expensive—anywhere from 25 to 200 percent—than "conventional" groceries. I have several thoughts on this:

1. Yes, organic foods are more expensive, but the taste and quality are far superior and much healthier for you and your family. Eating organic foods greatly reduces your exposure to chemicals and pesticides prevalent in conventionally produced food. You can also save money by purchasing organically grown produce in season at farmer's markets and roadside stands, which are often cheaper than the supermarket. (Be sure to ask if the fruits and vegetables are organic and pesticide-free.)

2. Eating organic food prepared at home is *cheaper* than taking the family to a fast-food stop like Burger King or a "fast casual" restaurant like Panera Bread. It's hard to get away for under $20 at a typical fast-food joint (for a family of four), and the tab is closer to $30 for two parents and two kids at a fast casual restaurant. Believe me, you could feed the family several scrumptious organic dinners, complete with grass-fed beef or wild-caught fish, for what it would cost to go out one evening at a quick-service restaurant. The family could dine an entire week on home-cooked organic food for the price of a sit-down meal at a well-appointed establishment with linen tablecloths, shiny silverware, and snooty waiters.

3. Eating organic food is less expensive than following a special diet or dietetic meal plan. *Forbes* magazine examined the weekly menus from the top ten most popular diets on the market: Atkins, Jenny Craig, Ornish, NutriSystem, Slim-Fast, South Beach, Subway (yes, the Jared diet of eating low-fat Subway sandwiches twice a day), Sugar Busters!, Weight Watchers, and Zone. A week's worth of Jenny Craig–supplied meals cost the most: $137.65 per week; the Subway

sandwich diet was the least expensive, at $68.90. But all ten diets were 50 percent more than the $54.44 that the average single American spends on food weekly.[3]

If losing weight or childhood obesity is an issue in your home, let me make one more point. The Seven Keys laid out in *The Great Physician's Rx for Women's Health* may not seem directly related to weight loss, but they are part of living a healthy lifestyle and will help you attain and maintain your ideal weight. Many people have told us that the Great Physician's prescription has helped them lose pounds that wouldn't come off with any other diet. In fact, at a recent Women of Faith conference, dozens of women approached Jordan and shared their phenomenal success stories, complete with a few tears of joy.

If you're looking for a total women's health plan that can help you shed those extra pounds, you've come to the right place, but if you're looking for even faster weight loss, I urge you to check out Jordan's book *The Great Physician's Rx for Weight Loss.*

Not only are organic foods tastier, but they also pack more nutritional punch, both in terms of dry weight and nutrients. *The Journal of Applied Nutrition,* over a two-year period, purchased both organically and conventionally grown apples, potatoes, pears, wheat, and sweet corn in the western suburbs of Chicago and analyzed these foods for their mineral contents. Four to fifteen samples were taken for each food group.

On a per-weight basis, average levels of essential minerals were much higher in organically grown versus conventionally grown food. The organically grown food averaged 63 percent higher in calcium, 78 percent higher in chromium, 118 percent higher in magnesium, 178 percent higher in molybdenum, 91 percent higher in phosphorus, 125 percent higher in potassium, and 60 percent higher in zinc. And one more thing: organically raised food averaged 29 percent lower in mercury—a toxin—than the conventionally raised food.[4]

"Organic foods" means much more than plump red tomatoes fresh from the vine versus the half-green kind grown under hothouse conditions and picked long before they're ripe. When I talk about organic foods, I'm referring to grains, dairy products, and meats, the latter coming from livestock that chew fresh grass in open fields or on organic feed that isn't laced with antibiotics and growth hormones to fatten them up for the slaughterhouse. Organic crops come from fields that haven't been doused with chemical pesticides, herbicides, and synthetic fertilizers, while conventionally grown crops are grown in tired soils that have lost much of their nutrient potency over the last hundred years because of rampant mineral depletion. The nutritive value of today's conventionally grown foods doesn't hold a candle to what our forebears ate.

In 2002, the U.S. Department of Agriculture set standards that producers and handlers must follow in order to be certified by the USDA as organic. To receive a "100% Organic" seal, the product must be all-organic, which means the fruit or vegetable was grown without the use of most synthetic and petroleum-derived pesticides and fertilizers, antibiotics, genetic engineering, irradiation, and sewer sludge for three consecutive years. Organic meats must come from animals that eat 100 percent organic feed, without animal by-products; and for dairy cows, the whole herd must have eaten organic feed for the past one-year period.[5] A USDA seal reading "Organic" means that the product is at least 95 percent organic, and "Made with Organic Ingredients" means at least 70 percent of the ingredients are organic.

Shopping for organic foods in health food or whole food stores provides the surest path to eating foods that God created. At the end of this chapter, I'll tell you the best foods to shop for and eat, but first, let's talk about optimizing nutrition, which begins with an awareness of what you're dropping into your shopping cart. To begin with, everything we eat is either a protein, a fat, or a carbohydrate. Let's take a closer look at these macronutrients.

## The Importance of Protein

Were you aware that proteins are necessary for building your muscles and maintaining good skin tone, healthy hair, strong nails, and virtually every other body part or tissue? Did you know that 75 percent of your weight—if you took away the water inside your body—is protein?[6] We need to eat proteins because they provide for the transportation of nutrients, oxygen, and waste throughout the body.

Proteins are comprised of various numbers and combinations of twenty-two amino acids that we need to live a robust life, but our bodies are incapable of producing all twenty-two. Scientists have discovered that eight essential amino acids are missing, meaning that they must come from the foods we eat. It just so happens that animal proteins—chicken, beef, lamb, dairy, eggs, and so on—are the only complete protein sources providing the Big Eight amino acids in their correct ratios.

Nutritionists recommend eating nine grams of protein for every twenty pounds of weight, or between sixty and seventy grams of protein per day. Though billions around the world wake up each morning without enough protein to eat, we don't have that problem in the U.S. Our problem is that we're not eating from the *best sources* of animal protein: organically raised cattle, sheep, goats, buffalo, venison, poultry, wild-caught fish, dairy, and eggs.

Grass-fed red meat is leaner and lower in calories than grain-fed. Organic beef is higher in heart-friendly omega-3 fatty acids and is an important source of vitamins, like $B_{12}$ and E. It is much better for you than steaks and burgers from hormone-injected cattle that chewed on pesticide-sprayed feed laced with antibiotics.

Fish with scales and fins, caught from oceans and rivers, are excellent sources of protein and provide the essential amino acids. The good news is that, in addition to natural food stores, fish markets, and specialty shops, these days supermarkets are making fresh, wild-caught fish available.

**Nicki:** Listen up, ladies: eating quality proteins supports weight loss. In the last few years, head-to-head comparison trials have shown that high-protein, low-carbohydrate diets seem more effective for weight loss than low-fat, high-carbohydrate diets, at least in the first six months, according to the Harvard School of Public Health.

Apparently, a high-protein diet with plenty of chicken, beef, fish, dairy, eggs, and other high-protein foods, along with the healthy fats they contain, slows the movement of food from the stomach to the intestine. Slower stomach emptying means you feel full for longer and get hungrier later. Second, protein has a gentle, steady effect on blood sugar as compared to the spike in blood sugar that you get after eating a rapidly digested carbohydrate food such as white bread or a baked potato.

**Jordan:** Choosing high-protein foods that contain healthy fats, such as omega-3s, will help the heart as it helps the waistline. But here's a word of caution: don't go overboard eating proteins to the exclusion of everything else. Avoiding fruits, vegetables, and whole grains means missing out on healthful fiber, vitamins, minerals, and other phytonutrients.

Now let's get the skinny on fats.

## Checking Out Fats

If you were a teenager during the 1990s, you probably read influential articles in *People* and *Parade* magazines about how bad fat was for you. These stories planted the notion that if you wanted to lose weight, then eating foods without fat would do the trick. Young girls took that advice to heart, believing that if they eliminated fat from their diets, they would be as thin as the supermodels taking flight down the runways of Milan and Paris. In a demonstration of the law of unintended circumstances, however, the result was an unprecedented leap in anorexia and bulimia among weight-conscious teen girls.

**Nicki:** I was a teenager back then, and I can remember this wacky woman with spiked platinum hair, named Susan Powter, who screamed at us to "stop the insanity" because "it's fat that's making you fat!" Girls in my high school nodded in agreement and gobbled up anything with the magic words "fat-free" or "reduced fat" on the packaging: cheese, crackers, cookies, yogurt, and ice cream. My friends studied salad-dressing labels as if they were the Dead Sea Scrolls, and they were obsessed with fat grams. I knew classmates who became borderline anorexic because of their fat phobia.

**Jordan:** Teen girls and young adult women were greatly influenced by a couple of best-selling diet books in the 1990s: *The Pritikin Principle* by Robert Pritikin and *Eat More, Weigh Less: Dr. Ornish's Program for Losing Weight Safely While Eating Abundantly* by Dean Ornish, MD, which preached the gospel of low-fat, high-carb diets. The Pritikin approach involved a diet based on vegetables and fruits, mostly raw, as well as whole grains and some meat. Pritikin advocated the elimination of sugar and white flour, which pretty much eliminated all processed foods. The Ornish diet was similar to Pritikin's but was close to vegan in its approach; the only animal products allowed were egg whites and one cup of nonfat milk or yogurt each day.

Pritikin and Ornish found adherents. Back in 1995, 44 percent of urban women were on a low-fat diet (as compared to 26 percent of urban men), according to the consumer research firm Decision Analyst, Inc.[7] Food manufacturers responded to this expanding market over the next decade by flooding supermarket aisles with thousands of low-fat and reduced-fat products. Restaurants revamped their menus with low-fat entrees to suit the changing tastes of health-conscious consumers.

Did low-fat blueberry muffins and reduced-fat ice cream make us any thinner? Not at all, especially if you take note of how we've become *fatter* as a nation since the mid-1990s. Every day, it seems, newspapers and news magazines publish breathless stories about the obesity "epidemic" threatening to destroy our nation.

### *The Genesis of Our Downfall*

This is our version of a cute story we once heard:

In the beginning, God created the heavens and the earth, and He populated the earth with green, yellow, and red vegetables, fruits of all kinds, seeds and grains, and healthy animals to provide meat and dairy products, all so that Man and Woman could live long and healthy lives.

Then, using God's great gifts, Satan created ice cream and glazed doughnuts. And Satan said to Man, "You want chocolate with that?" And Man replied, "Yes!" and Woman said, "As long as you're at it, add some sprinkles." Man and Woman gained ten pounds, and Satan smiled.

Then God created healthful yogurt so that Woman might keep the figure that Man found so fair. But Satan brought forth white flour from the wheat, and sugar from the cane, and he combined them. And Woman went from a size 6 to a size 14.

So God said, "Try my fresh green salad," and Satan presented Thousand Island dressing, greasy croutons, bacon bits, and white rolls on the side. And Man and Woman unfastened their belts following the repast.

God then said, "I have sent you heart-healthy vegetables, cold-water fish, and cold-pressed oils in which to cook them." But Satan brought forth deep-fried breaded fish, French fries, and hush puppies. So Man and Woman gained more weight, and their cholesterol levels went through the roof.

God then created whole-grain pasta that was thin and delicious, and He called it angel hair, topped it with organic tomato sauce, and declared, "It is good." Satan then created chocolate cake and named it "Devil's Food."

God then brought forth running shoes so that His children might lose those extra pounds. But Satan gave them cable TV with a remote control so Man would not have to toil changing the channels. And Man and Woman laughed and cried before the flickering blue light and gained another twenty pounds.

Then God brought forth the potato, naturally brimming with nutrition. But Satan peeled off the healthful skin and sliced the starchy center into chips and deep-fried them in shortening. And Man and Woman gained another ten pounds.

God then gave grass-fed beef, rich in iron and zinc and low in fat, so that Man and Woman might consume more minerals and fewer calories and still satisfy their appetites. But Satan created fast-food restaurants and ninety-nine-cent double cheeseburgers. Then he said, "You want fries with that?"

"Yes! And supersize them!" Man replied.

Satan said, "It is good," and Man went into cardiac arrest.

God sighed and created quadruple bypass surgery.

And then Satan created HMOs.

What happened is that all those low-fat diets had several things working against them. First, most people could not stay on them for any length of time, especially teen girls in the throes of adolescence and hormonal changes. In addition, "Those who possessed enough willpower to remain fat-free for any length of time developed a variety of health problems including low energy, difficulty in concentration, depression, weight gain, and mineral deficiencies," wrote Mary Enig, PhD, and Sally Fallon in *Nourishing Traditions.*[8]

In my view, low-fat diets failed to distinguish between the so-called "good fats" in food (including olive and flaxseed; tropical oils, such as coconut oil; and fish oils) and the "bad fats" (hydrogenated oils found in margarine and most packaged goods) associated with clogged arteries, heart disease, and other health problems. We need certain fats in our diet to provide a concentrated source of energy and source material for cell membranes and various hormones. The fats we *don't* need are mainly hydrogenated and partially hydrogenated fats found in processed foods, which, as I've already mentioned, are what meals are built around these days. I'm talking about frosted flakes for breakfast, a glazed doughnut at break, fried corn chips and chocolate chip cookies for lunch, and breaded chicken nuggets for dinner.

When we prepare food these days, we may not reach for a tub of Crisco, as our moms may have done two decades ago, but we usually pour safflower, corn, or soybean oil (any of which may be partially hydrogenated) into the pan. In the process of hydrogenation, hydrogen gas is injected into the oil under high pressure to make the oil solid at room temperature, which prevents the oil from becoming rancid too quickly. Nice thought, but adulterating the oil carries a price since the hydrogenation process produces trans-fatty acids, also known as *trans fat.*

Trans fat has recently become a household term since the Food and Drug Administration, beginning in 2006, required new Nutritional Facts labels on all foods to state the amount of trans fat. I chuckled when I heard that several giant companies had quietly changed the composition of their foods rather than reveal that their popular foods were loaded with trans fat. Others

"reformulated" their products to remove trans fat bef
2006, labeling deadline.

Kraft Foods, which gave the world Velveeta Cheese—y
the look on Nicki's face during our dating days when I
Velveeta wasn't real cheese—reduced the trans fat content on *650* products by reformulating their makeups. When items such as Kraft Easy Mac, DiGiorno Thin Crispy Crust Pizza, original Oreo cookies, and Wheat Thins crackers reported "0 gram" trans fat per serving, the news was trumpeted in the media.[9]

Don't fall for the hype. While I'm happy that the feet of food companies are being held to the fire regarding trans fat, at the end of the day these products will never be as good as the foods God created. In case you're wondering, God created some wonderful fats that benefit the body and aid metabolism. Extra-virgin coconut oil, extra-virgin olive oil, and flaxseed oil, as well as almonds, avocados, and organically produced butter contain the fats you want to include in your diet; I urge you to stock your cupboard with these foods.

Extra-virgin coconut oil is excellent for cooking scrambled eggs or heating up leftovers. Use extra-virgin olive oil when making homemade salad dressing and as a great addition to warm foods *after* they've been cooked. I do not recommend it be used in cooking since certain nutrients break down under high heat.

## Carbohydrates

I believe Susan Powter had it all wrong: eating fat is not the reason people get fat. Eating foods with *excess* carbohydrates, especially processed foods, is often the culprit for jiggly tummies and padded thighs these days.

After the low-fat diets ran their course, mass-market women's magazines like *Redbook* and *McCall's* were searching high and low for the next get-thin-quick idea. The editors at the these major women's magazines—which are published in New York City—begin the day by reading the *New York Times*, which is one reason why "the Gray Lady," as the newspaper is called in the Big Apple, is so influential.

Their eyes certainly caught a major story in the *New York Times Magazine*, published on Sunday morning, July 7, 2002. In an article titled "What If It's All Been a Big Fat Lie?" reporter Gary Taubes wrote that the American medical establishment had been ridiculing Robert Atkins, a Manhattan cardiologist, for thirty years regarding his book, *The Atkins Diet Revolution* (originally released in 1972, and revised and released in 1992 as *The Atkins New Diet Revolution*). Dr. Atkins's best-selling books extolled the benefits of a low-carbohydrate, high-protein, high-fat diet, informing readers that increasing their intake of protein from meat, fish, and dairy, and reducing their intake of carbohydrates like bread, pasta, and rice, would reduce insulin levels and cause their bodies to burn excess body fat for fuel. A high-protein diet, very high in fat and very low in carbohydrates, he said, would lead to decreased appetite, lower food consumption, and weight loss.

Reporter Taubes declared that American doctors who recommended eating *less* fat and *more* carbohydrates—in other words, the low-fat diets—were the cause of the raging obesity epidemic in America, not level-headed folks like Dr. Atkins. The way things were turning out, "the unrepentant Atkins was right all along," Taubes declared. Much of his piece praised Dr. Atkins as a prophet whose voice needed to be heard, not banished to the wilderness.

The article set off a media stampede. Suddenly, pro-Atkins diet stories were everywhere. Editors and producers, who don't want to miss a bandwagon before it rolls out of town, assigned writers to come up with a series of fawning features. The major networks' news magazine shows fell like dominoes: NBC's *Dateline*, CBS's *48 Hours*, and ABC's *20/20* each ran their own stories on the virtues of an Atkins low-carb diet. Before you could say, "cheeseburger," *The Atkins New Diet Revolution* catapulted to number one on the *New York Times* best seller list. Today, the Atkins diet books have sold more than 45 million copies.[10]

In case you were living in a cave at the time, the Atkins diet was big on fried pork rinds, heavy cream, cheese, and meat. Dr. Atkins didn't have much good to say about bread and bananas, which he labeled as "poison" in his book. A typical Atkins diet breakfast is fried eggs and bacon; no toast, no cereal, no milk. Lunch is typically a chicken breast with melted mozzarella and mixed lettuce, and dinner might be something like a pan-fried steak with spinach. If you get the munchies before going to bed, then snack on a couple of pieces of ham.

When *The Atkins New Diet Revolution* rocketed to number one, low-carb was hotter than a day at Miami Beach—which happened to be the hometown of cardiologist Dr. Arthur Agatston, who had developed a low-carb diet plan to help his heart patients lose weight. *The South Beach Diet* was released in April 2003 and flew off the shelves as well.

Just as a rising tide lifts all boats, another low-carb diet book—this one originally published in the mid-1990s—found an audience. *The Zone,* written by research scientist Barry Sears, also became a best seller, though readers found its meal plans to be as complicated as a Rubik's Cube. If you followed Barry Sears's meal plans to the letter, you ate certain protein blocks, carbohydrate blocks, and fat blocks at each meal, but you had to eat these blocks every 4.5 hours—which amounted to eating five times per day—to remain in "the zone."

The low-carb craze peaked in early 2004, when more than 9 percent of U.S. adults claimed to be on a low-carb diet, according to market research firm NPD Group. That figure had declined to 2.2 percent a little more than a year later, the same time Atkins Nutritionals, the company distributing Atkins products, announced that it was seeking bankruptcy protection.[11]

It doesn't surprise me that the low-carb boom fizzled since the only good thing about low-carb diets was that people avoided excess sugar and white flour. Though each of the aforementioned diets has some good recommendations, I disagree with Atkins, South Beach, and the Zone approaches because they call for the excessive consumption of meats that the Bible calls detestable or unclean (I'll explain shortly). These diets also support the intake of processed foods loaded with chemicals and recommend the use of artificial sweeteners (Atkins and South Beach), though followers are allowed to eat a limited amount of nutrient-rich fruits and vegetables in the initial phases.

At the same time, however, I concede that there are some things I like about a lower-carbohydrate approach to eating, especially if you're trying to lose those excess pounds that have crept onto your frame. The standard

American diet is weighted way too heavily on the carb side, especially when you consider how many of our foods contain sugar. Read the labels on boxes and packages, and you'll find sugar, corn syrup, fructose, and sucrose to be among the first ingredients listed in cereals, breads, buns, pastries, doughnuts, cookies, ketchup, and ice cream.

Replacing these processed foods with natural and organic foods and consuming carbohydrates such as fruits, vegetables, nuts, seeds, legumes, and cultured dairy products —foods that are lower calorie, high in nutrients, and low in sugar— play an important part in losing weight and staying healthy.

Whether you need to lose a few inches or you're just interested in eating and serving the healthiest, most nutritious food possible, the following are Top Healing Foods that should find a way into your pantry or refrigerator:

• **Fermented dairy products.** Yogurt, kefir, raw hard cheeses, cottage cheese, and cultured cream are healthy foods that provide an easily absorbable form of naturally acidified calcium, which helps build strong bones in children and slows the development of osteoporosis, which is the bane of many women as they leave middle age. These cultured dairy products lower blood pressure and cholesterol levels while giving you an energy boost. The fermentation process makes the milk easier to digest and its nutrients more usable by the body.

High-quality fermented dairy can come from cow's milk, sheep's milk, or goat's milk. When moms reach for milk gallons in the supermarket dairy case, they often choose the 2% reduced fat or skim milk versions because they've been told to reduce saturated fat in their diets. Contrary to the prevailing conventional wisdom, however, I recommend the full-fat version because removing the fat makes the milk less nutritious and less digestible. After all, who's ever heard of a cow, sheep, or goat giving low-fat or fat-free milk?

Unfortunately, today's commercially available milk, which has been both pasteurized and homogenized, presents some health challenges. Reading William Campbell Douglass's *The Milk Book*, which makes a strong case for drinking raw certified milk instead of homogenized, pasteurized milk, has heavily influenced me. Unfortunately, raw certified milk is not widely available, thanks to the "Got Milk?" lobby and the National Dairy Council. If you can't find certified raw milk, then cultured or fermented dairy products, such as yogurt and kefir (which is produced from pasteurized, nonhomogenized milk), are the next best thing because they are excellent sources of easily digestible protein, B vitamins, calcium, and probiotics. If raw milk is unavailable, it's best to choose pasteurized—but nonhomogenized—milk, which is usually contained in glass bottles at your health food store.

Goat's milk is naturally homogenized and is a good alternative for those allergic to cow's milk and who don't tolerate soy milk well. It is less allergenic because it does not contain the same complex proteins found in cow's milk. Goat's milk is an acquired taste, but I prefer its molecular structure: its fat and protein molecules are tiny in size, which allows for rapid absorption in the digestive tract.

• **Red meat.** Many women have clinical or subclinical iron deficiency anemia. A Penn State University study showed that iron-deficient women performed significantly worse on memory and attention tests than healthy women, and they experienced fatigue and irritability.[12]

Eating red meat in the form of sustainably raised beef, bison, lamb, goat, or venison is an excellent way to build up iron in your bloodstream, especially the week after menstruation, when you lose a good amount of blood. You'll be much better off purchasing meats that are organically raised or designated as grass-fed or open-pastured. I recommend grass-fed or pastured beef, lamb, bison, and venison because these meats are naturally leaner and contain large concentrations of nutrients and healthy fats. In addition, grass-fed, natural meats are free from chemicals and hormones.

• **Wild-caught fish.** Fish caught in the wild, instead of those raised on fish farms, provide a richer source of omega-3 fat, protein, vitamins, and minerals. It's getting easier to shop for salmon these days because U.S. supermarkets have been required to label salmon as farmed or wild. Line-caught fish from Alaska are the healthiest to eat since their habitats are more pristine in the forty-ninth state. If you see a package marked "Atlantic salmon," you can figure that those were farm-raised. Feedlot salmon can't compare to their cold-water cousins in terms of taste or nutritional value because they spend their days cooped up in concrete tanks, swimming in circles as they wait for the next shovelful of food pellets to be tossed their way.

• **Canned salmon, sardines, and low-mercury, high omega-3 tuna.** Though any fish is a good source of calcium, canned wild salmon and sardines are particularly high in omega-3 fatty acids and calcium. Don't be squeamish about eating a few bones—they are actually soft and quite edible—since they contain calcium phosphate and fluoride. These tiny fish are also a good source of selenium, which helps to protect cells from damage by acting as an antioxidant.

Canned tuna, which has long been the darling of the weight conscious, has been the subject of much disdain due to high levels of heavy metals, including mercury. There is now available a low-mercury, high omega-3 tuna that is extremely healthy and safe to consume a few cans per week. (For recommended brands, visit www.BiblicalHealthInstitute.com and click on the GPRx Resource Guide.)

Be careful about eating conventional canned tuna, which can raise your exposure to mercury. Conventional tuna consumption should be limited to two or three cans per week and not more than a can per week—or not at all—if you are pregnant. Best to err on the side of safety when your body is nurturing a growing baby.

• **Nuts and seeds.** Walnuts and flaxseeds are high in omega-3 fatty acids. Almonds and black sesame seeds are high in calcium, but soak these first so they will be easier to digest. Place them in a bowl, add one teaspoon of salt, and cover them with water for six to eight hours. Then drain the water and place the nuts or seeds on a cookie sheet to dry on low heat in the oven.

Nuts and seeds contain indigestible remnants of fiber, or "roughage." These foods can help you stay regular and avoid constipation.

• **Leafy greens high in magnesium.** These include spinach and heads of romaine, red leaf, and butterhead lettuce, as well as the less nutritious crisp-head, or iceberg, lettuce. (Generally speaking, the darker green the leaves, the more nutritious the salad will be.) These green foods contain a broad array of enzymes, vitamins, minerals, proteins, and chlorophyll, the green pigment found in plants. The main element in chlorophyll is magnesium, and every cell in your body needs it, as it performs more than three hundred biochemical reactions in the body.[13] Bone health, for example, is greatly improved by the magnesium contained in greens. By eating leafy green salads regularly, your body receives the magnesium it needs.

We have no excuse to not eat healthy salads year-round. Due to improved shipping and storage methods, lettuce is one of the most widely available fresh vegetables. We buy the organic, prewashed green lettuce blends: mix in some carrots, cucumber, red onions, and red peppers; add a healthy salad dressing; and you get your magnesium while dining on some of the healthiest foods on the planet.

Without enough magnesium in the blood, hearts beat irregularly, arteries stiffen, blood pressure rises, blood tends to clot, muscles spasm, insulin grows weaker, bones lose strength, and pain signals intensify.[14] These are powerful reasons to eat plenty of salad, preferably organic, since it's likely to have greater concentrations of magnesium.

• **Fruits and veggies.** Eating plenty of fruits and vegetables, especially during your menstrual cycle, helps women naturally cleanse their bodies. Many vegetables are high in calcium, magnesium, and potassium, which help relieve and prevent muscle spasms during your period. Tori Hudson, author of *Women's Encyclopedia of Natural Medicine,* points out that fruits are an excellent source of natural anti-inflammatory substances such as bioflavonoids and vitamin C. "These nutrients not only strengthen the blood vessels that aid circulation to areas of muscle tension in the pelvis but also reduce the pain from menstrual cramps through their anti-inflammatory effect," she wrote.[15]

*The Encyclopedia of Natural Healing* relates that by upping your consumption of green vegetables, you can avoid calcium deficiency and prevent menstrual cramps.[16] Complex carbohydrates such as whole grains, beans, fresh fruit, and vegetables may also help relieve premenstrual symptoms. You may want to back off of animal protein for a few days leading up to the start of your period and go for complex carbs instead.

## *Had a Yeast Infection Yet?*

*by Pancheta Wilson, MD*

It is normal for a few yeast cells to exist in the vagina, though there is usually a balance between the good bacteria and disease-causing organisms such as yeast. But when this balance is disturbed for any reason, it sets the stage for an overgrowth of yeast and other organisms, which is not uncommon. The U.S. National Women's Health Information Center estimates that 75 percent of women will suffer an irritation of the vagina and vulva due to yeast overgrowth sometime during their lives.[17] And because the urethra is in close proximity to the vagina and the anus, where harmful bacteria abound, there is a predisposition to concurrent infection of the vagina and the urinary tract.

Yeast infections can make lovemaking very uncomfortable and even painful. Urination may be accompanied by a stinging or burning sensation. Candida overgrowth in the gut can have systemic and local effects, such as hormonal, skin, and immune system disorders. (If you suspect candida excess, or other infections, seek the help of a physician. Meanwhile, a simple questionnaire at www.yeastconnection.com/yeast.html can help you evaluate the role yeast plays in your chronic health problems.)

The major cause of candida overgrowth leading to vaginal infection is the overuse of oral antibiotics. Other contributing factors include changes in the body's pH balance, dehydration, improper use of antacids, and oral contraceptives (oral contraceptives do not cause yeast infections but make them more difficult to treat). Diabetes and other conditions that suppress the immune system are also associated with frequent yeast and bacterial infections. Both the U.S. government and most physicians seem unaware that foods containing sugar and white flour can contribute to these types of infections.

If you have a vaginal yeast infection, try to avoid taking potent prescription and over-the-counter antifungal agents as much as possible, since these drugs can be harmful to the liver and the immune system. I recommend changing your diet as outlined in the *Great Physician's Rx for Women's Health* as your first step in dealing with this issue.

William Crook, MD, author of *The Yeast Connection and Women's Health*, said that without changes in diet, "You won't get the results you're hoping for." His yeast-fighting diet calls for organic meats and fish, fresh vegetables, healthy fats, nuts, seeds, and pure water—foods part of the Great Physician's prescription for women's health. I'm confident that candida overgrowth can be mitigated by adding probiotic-rich foods like yogurt and kefir, as well as raw sauerkraut, to your diet. Dr. Crook recommends the elimination of sugar and yeast from your diet for at least three weeks—and sometimes longer.

Dr. Crook, who died in 2002, made it his life mission to study and treat yeast infections. He believed there was a connection between the systemic overgrowth of *Candida albicans* (yeast) and premenstrual syndrome (PMS), so if you know that you get a little crazy just before your time of the month, don't delay in eating healthy foods that God created for your body.

• **Fermented veggies.** It may be impossible to get your kids to try fermented vegetables, such as cucumbers, sauerkraut, beets, or pickled carrots, but don't let that stop you from giving these vitamin- and mineral-packed foods a try. Fermented vegetables contain friendly microorganisms known as *probiotics*, as well as concentrated amounts of vitamins, including vitamin C. If you're not a big sauerkraut or pickled-beet fan, try adding pickled relish atop broiled fish. Fermented foods are effective in releasing important nutritional compounds during the predigestive phase of the digestion process.

• **Fermented soy.** I know I've been recommending a lot of fermented foods, but the fermentation process is the oldest known form of food biotechnology, dating back thousands of years. Fermentation enriches food in terms of protein, essential amino acids, essential fatty acids, vitamins, carbohydrates, and assorted antioxidants.

Fermented soy products, such as miso, tempeh, natto, and brewed soy sauce, have their roots in the Far East, where traditional fermented soy foods are considered to have significant health-promoting benefits. Fermented soy products have been shown to help ease the uncomfortable symptoms associated with menopause, including hot flashes, night sweats, vaginal dryness, irritability, and bone loss. The next time you visit a health food store, check out these foods and give them a try.

• **Beta glucans from soluble oat fiber.** Beta glucans are a class of nondigestive polysaccharides—meaning they are relatively complex carbohydrates—widely found in oats, barley, and yeast. They are noted for their ability to enhance the immune system and promote healthy blood sugar and cholesterol levels. A good way to introduce beta glucans into your system is to consume whole food nutrition bars and meal replacement shakes containing the recommended daily amount of beta glucans from soluble oat fiber. (For recommended brands, visit www.BiblicalHealthInstitute.com and click on the GPRx Resource Guide.)

• **Water, tea, and coffee.** These beverages are not foods, but from what Nicki tells me, most women don't drink the amount of water they should because they fear they'll have to go to the bathroom too often. Let me encourage you to drink plenty of water anyway because this remarkable resource performs so many vital tasks for the body: regulating body temperature, carrying nutrients and oxygen to the cells, cushioning joints, protecting organs and tissues, and removing toxins from the body.

How much water should one drink? A good rule of thumb for minimum hydration is a half ounce of water for every pound of body weight, and an additional 16 ounces of water per hour of exercise. So Nicki, who weighs 110 pounds, should drink 55 ounces of water a day when she doesn't exercise and 71 ounces when she exercises for an hour (seven to nine 8-ounce glasses of water a day).

Some women think that if they drink that much water, they'll gain weight because they'll "retain" water. Unless there is an underlying medical problem, the opposite occurs. If you're trying to lose weight, you want to drink *more* water than ever before because drinking fluids both flushes out toxins in the digestive tract *and* dampens late morning and late afternoon hunger pangs. Drinking a glass of water ten to thirty minutes before mealtime will take the edge off of stomach growls and give you less of a reason to raid the fridge or pillage the pantry.

F. Batmanghelidj, MD, and author of *You're Not Sick, You're Thirsty!*, contends that you'll lose weight if you drink a glass of water thirty minutes before you eat and two glasses two and a half hours later. "You will feel full and will eat only when food is needed," he says. "The volume of food intake will decrease drastically. The type of cravings for food will also change. With sufficient water intake, we tend to crave proteins more than carbohydrates. If you think you are different and your body does not need eight to ten glasses of water each day, you are making a major mistake," notes Dr. Batmanghelidj,[18] who believes that many women confuse hunger with thirst, thinking they're hungry when actually they're dehydrated.

Please note that as women age, they are prone to dehydration, so make sure you stay ahead of the curve and drink enough water. One way to know if you're drinking enough water is by looking at the color of your urine. If your urine is consistently yellow, you're not drinking enough water. Clear or light yellow urine is the best indicator that you're properly hydrated.

Don't overlook teas and herbal infusions, which can increase energy, enhance the immune system, improve digestion, and even help you wind down after a long day. I recommend a cup of hot tea and honey with breakfast, dinner, and snacks, but you can also drink freshly made iced tea. Please note that tea cannot be substituted for water. While tea provides many great health benefits, nothing can replace pure water for hydration. You can safely and healthfully consume two to four cups of tea and herbal infusions daily, but you still need at least eight glasses of pure water.

As surprising as this may seem, coffee can be healthy if consumed the right way: without nondairy creamer and refined sugar or artificial sweeteners. I believe that coffee, which is high in antioxidants, should be made from freshly ground organic beans and stirred with your choice of the following: organic honey, unrefined sugar, a small amount of nonhomogenized organic milk, or heavy cream. Coffee consumption should be limited to one cup per day. (Caffeine is OK in small amounts, but it happens to be one of the most widely abused "drugs" in America.)

• **Fasting.** I know I've been talking a lot about eating and drinking, but another important part of a healthy lifestyle is giving the body's digestive system some time to kick back and relax, i.e., fasting. I know what you're thinking: *When do I ever get a chance to relax?*

You may feel that fasting is the *last* thing you have the energy to attempt, but let me propose something realistic that may work for you: a one-day *partial* fast, once a week. Skip breakfast and lunch, and eat dinner with the family. An eighteen- or twenty-hour respite from food delivers immediate benefits: you'll feel great when you come off the fast, you'll flush out toxins stored in your body (they tend to accumulate in the abdominal area), you'll lose weight, you'll gain time to accomplish more things, and you'll get closer to the Lord.

There's something about denying food to your body that increases your ability to hear what God has to say to you. Fasting and prayer go hand in hand, and I promise that you'll experience a renewed sense of well-being when you fast and give your hunger to Him. Arthur Wallis, author of *God's Chosen Fast,* says that fasting, when exercised with a pure heart and a right motive, may provide a key to unlock doors where other keys have failed, a spiritual weapon mighty enough to pull down strongholds.

When beginning a fast in the morning, start with a quiet time of reflection and reading some of your favorite Psalms. If you close your eyes and pray, don't be surprised if the Lord directs you to a certain section or verse of Scripture. Many people feel they hear God's voice more clearly in the midst of a fast.

A good place to read about fasting in Scripture is Isaiah 58, where the prophet teaches that fasting encourages humility, loosens the chains of injustice, and motivates us to treat others as we want to be treated. The heart of this chapter's message is contained in verses 6, 8, and 9:

> Is this not the [kind of] fast that I have chosen: to loose the bonds of wickedness, to undo the heavy burdens, to let the oppressed go free, and that you break every yoke? . . . Then your light shall break forth like the morning, your healing shall spring forth speedily; and your righteousness shall go before you; the glory of the LORD will be your rear guard. Then you shall call, and the LORD will answer; you shall cry, and He will say, "Here I am." (NKJV)

After you've had a time of reading Scripture, write down prayer requests on a piece of paper or in a journal, which is a tangible expression of dependence upon the Lord. Throughout the day, as hunger pains arise, think of one or more of those prayer requests as you lift up your needs to God.

Maintain a normal schedule, drinking only water or raw juices at room temperature since ice-cold beverages will shock the stomach. Lukewarm liquids will flush toxins from your body and satiate some of the hunger pains. And make sure to have plenty to do while fasting (as though you don't!) so the hours pass quickly. I tend to fast on Thursdays or Fridays since the weekend is coming up, and dropping a pound or two before any social events is never a bad thing.

When breaking a fast, don't start with a heavy meat-and-potatoes, pass-the-gravy meal. A large green salad, chicken or beef broth, and some raw, fermented veggies is an excellent way to resume eating.

*Something to Chew On*
*by Jordan Rubin*

As a culture, we eat too fast, but that's what happens when you eat on the run. For some folks, eating is nothing more than a pit stop; we all know people who mindlessly munch on something as they perform some other task, like ironing or cleaning up around the house.

Though I'm no "foodie," whose idea of a good time is sitting down to a two-hour lunch followed by a three-hour dinner, I'm well aware of the physiological importance of sitting down and calmly, thoroughly chewing my food before swallowing. That's why I recommend chewing each mouthful of food twenty-five to seventy-five times before gulping and swallowing. This advice may sound ridiculous, but a conscious effort to chew slowly ensures that plenty of digestive juices are added to the food before it begins to wind its way through the digestive tract.

Chewing food properly allows enzymes in your saliva to turn the food into a near-liquid form before swallowing. The act of working your jaw also sends a neurological message to your stomach and pancreas to increase acid and digestive enzyme production because food's on the way. This is especially important when eating foods high in starches and sugars since *ptyalin*, a salivary enzyme, helps break down these foods.

Chewing your food well can also significantly reduce postmeal bloating. If you chew your food longer, the brain will receive a signal that you're getting full, so you will feel satisfied earlier, eat less, and experience fewer digestive problems.

## THE DIRTY DOZEN: FOODS TO AVOID

**Jordan:** So far we've talked about the best foods to eat, but I've also come up with a list of "Dirty Dozen" foods that should never find a way onto your dinner table:

1. **Pork products.** In all of my books, I've consistently pointed out that pork should be avoided because God called pigs "detestable" or "unclean" in the Old Testament. We'll explain in greater detail in the next section beginning on page 31.
2. **Shellfish, and fish without fins and scales, such as catfish, shark, and eel.** God also called hard-shelled crustaceans, such as lobsters, crabs, and clams, unclean.
3. **Hydrogenated oils.** Sorry, Crisco lovers, but don't cook with shortening or margarine, which contain unhealthy fats. Also avoid processed

chips, crackers, and other baked goods, which often contain hydrogenated oils.

4. **Artificial sweeteners.** Aspartame, saccharin, sucralose, and its sweet cousins are made from chemicals that have sparked debate for decades. Though the Food and Drug Administration has approved the use of artificial sweeteners in drinks and food, these chemical additives may prove to be detrimental to your health in the long term. H. J. Roberts, MD, an authority on artificial sweeteners, testified at congressional hearings that artificial sweeteners can be highly addictive and trigger toxic substances to cross the blood-brain barrier, causing neurological problems.[19]

5. **White flour.** Enriched flour, which has been stripped during the milling process of half of the healthy fatty acids and fiber, as well as the wheat germ and bran, is the main ingredient in bread, bagels, rolls, and buns. The healthy alternative—whole-wheat bread made from unprocessed whole-grain flour—is a lot healthier and easy to find these days.

6. **White sugar.** If you're looking for a culprit to blame for increased pant sizes, look no farther. Many people don't realize that they eat sugar all day long: from breakfast cereal to flavored coffees to snack cookies to à la mode desserts. Sugar consumption can also have a deleterious effect on the immune system.

7. **Soft drinks.** These are nothing more than liquefied sugar. A 12-ounce can of Coke or Pepsi is the equivalent of eating nearly nine teaspoons of sugar. On a per capita basis, we drink 460 soft drinks per person each year; that's more than one Coke or Pepsi per day and 69,000 calories per year![20] Soft drinks are also high in phosphoric acid, which is detrimental to bone health.

8. **Pasteurized, homogenized skim milk.** Goat's milk is good; whole, organic nonhomogenized milk is better; and cultured whole-milk dairy, like yogurt and kefir, is better still.

9. **Corn syrup.** This version of sugar is even more fattening.

10. **Hydrolyzed soy protein.** If you're wondering what in the world this is, hydrolyzed soy protein is found in imitation meat products and other processed foods and is a known *excitotoxin*, which means it has the potential to cause neurological disturbances.

11. **Artificial flavors and colors.** It seems as if every food pitched to kids is made with artificial flavors and colors. These additives can contribute to behavioral problems in children and increase the body's toxic load, and they are associated with allergies and skin rashes.

12. **Excessive alcohol.** Long-term, excessive drinking damages every organ in the body (especially the liver), adds weight, produces heart problems, promotes depression, causes digestive ailments (ulcers, gastritis, and pancreatitis), and impacts fertility.

*Is Chocolate a Woman's Best Friend?*
*by Nicki Rubin*

About a month after Jordan and I started dating, Valentine's Day arrived. I'll never forget when he dropped by my apartment and presented me with a heart-shaped box of chocolates. I wasn't a candy eater—remember, I was the healthiest person I knew—but I appreciated the sentiments behind the thoughtful gift. I opened the box to find seven pieces of chocolate, each foil-wrapped, in the shape of a heart.

"It's organic chocolate," he explained. "They said at the health food store that it's the best kind."

"Would you like a piece?" I asked, holding the box in front of me.

"No, I couldn't. I'm not eating any chocolate, but you go right ahead."

We sat down next to each other on the couch. I looked at each piece carefully before choosing one. After unwrapping the red foil, I popped it into my mouth. Incredible! I had never eaten chocolate that tasted so good before!

I didn't stop with one piece, or two. Nor three or four. I ate the *whole* box of chocolate in one sitting. "These are fantastic," I said between gooey bites.

Nine years later, I'm still not much of a candy eater, and I understand that white sugar is terribly unhealthy to eat, but I still have a weakness for chocolate. To quote model Claudia Schiffer, "Once in a while I say, 'Go for it,' and I eat chocolate."

Women have been going for chocolate for a long time. Maybe it has something to do with our monthly hormonal cycles. It's believed that Christopher Columbus brought back the first cocoa beans from the New World in 1502, and the first chocolate bar was produced in 1828, when Conrad Van Houten, a Dutch chemist, invented a cocoa press that mixed cocoa butter with finely ground sugar. "Chocolate is no ordinary food," writer Geneen Roth explains. "It is not something you can take or leave, something you like only moderately. You don't like chocolate. You don't even love chocolate. Chocolate is something you have an affair with."[21]

Well, I wouldn't go that far, but chocolate is delicious and can even be healthy—in small doses. Dark chocolate, preferably made from organic ingredients, is better for you than lighter milk chocolate because it's higher in healthy bioflavanoids, an antioxidant. Dark chocolate also releases both serotonin and endorphins, which act as antidepressants.[22]

Furthermore, chocolate contains a high level of phenylethylamine, the same chemical that the brain produces when you fall in love. I wonder if Jordan knew that when he brought me that box of organic chocolate on Valentine's Day . . .

### WHIRLWIND TRIP

**Nicki:** Our hosts, Mike and Nicole Yorkey, called it "Three Meals, Three Countries."

"We'll have breakfast in France, lunch in Italy, and dinner in Switzerland," Nicole explained. Her husband, Mike, helps Jordan with the research, writing, and editing of his books, and they had invited us to Switzerland, where Nicole grew up before coming to the United States at age twenty-one to teach skiing.

(She met Mike at Mammoth Mountain in California's Eastern Sierra mountains, where she was teaching ski classes.)

Nicole's idea sounded great to me, so during our Swiss trip in the fall of 2005, we motored to picturesque Annecy, France, about two hours from their family chalet in Villars, Switzerland. The next morning, we were served a typical European continental breakfast—croissants, artisan breads, cereal, and fruit—at our cute hotel tucked away in the cobblestone-paved and car-free Vieux Ville, or Old Town, while Jordan chose to eat whole-milk yogurt, honey, and fruit. Afterward, the four of us took a leisurely boat ride around the glassy Lake of Annecy, the "purest lake in Europe," if I understood the guide's heavily accented English correctly.

In the early afternoon, we hopped in our four-door Renault and drove into the massive Alpine region known as the Haute Savoie, where we paid $40 to drive a seven-mile tunnel cut through the bedrock of the Mont Blanc, Europe's tallest peak. Within minutes, we saw the light at the end of the tunnel, which meant that we were in Italy. There we strolled through Aosta's pedestrian-only downtown, amid densely packed buildings oozing with Roman charm and streets as old as Caesar. Our stomachs were growling by midafternoon; everyone was famished. We eyed a pizzeria and took a seat at an outdoor table.

Let's just say that the *menu turistico* wasn't inscribed in English. Nicole, who speaks excellent Italian (as well as four other languages), scanned the *carta* and patiently explained the kinds of pizza we could order: there was *pizza con prosciutto di Parma, pizza con crude, pizza con culatello* . . . When I asked Nicole to translate, she said that every pizza was topped with ham—raw (yuck!), cooked, cured, or smoked. That wasn't going to work for me because I hadn't eaten pork since 1998. It was a "detestable" animal that God had clearly said not to eat in Leviticus 11 and Deuteronomy 14. Rex Russell, MD, author of *What the Bible Says About Healthy Living*, had this to say about the perils of pork:

> One reason for God's rule forbidding pork is that the digestive system of a pig is completely different from that of a cow. It is similar to ours, in that the stomach is very acidic. Their stomach acids become diluted because of the

> volume of food, allowing all kinds of vermin to pass through this protective barrier. Parasites, bacteria, viruses, and toxins can pass into the pig's flesh because of overeating. These toxins and infectious agents can be passed on to humans when they eat a pig's flesh.[23]

After reading about all the parasitic diseases that pigs unwittingly pass on to humans—trichinosis, wire worms, tapeworms, etc.—I could absolutely never eat pork again. As Jordan says in his seminars, "Eating rule number one: Don't eat anything that Jesus cast demons into!" (See Mark 5:2–15.)

Shellfish are taboo as well. The flesh of shrimp, crabs, lobsters, oysters, and clams contains concentrations of toxins because these shellfish are bottom-feeders that feed on fish droppings and the dregs of sea life. Shellfish do clean up the water, but whatever they consume goes straight into their systems and, eventually, their flesh. (Here's another one of Jordan's memorable sayings: "You've all heard that you are what you eat, but when it comes to animal food, you are what *they* ate!")

Ever since I was a little girl, I had wondered why we ate pork or shellfish when God said not to in the Bible. When an older man from church patted my head and said, "We don't have to go by that now," I shrugged my ten-year-old shoulders because every Christian I knew back then didn't think twice about ordering a massive mound of pork barbecue at San Antonio's restaurant after church. After falling in love with Jordan and hearing how he felt about the matter, I knew better.

Jordan was raised in a Messianic Jewish home, where pork was anathema. He grew up without ham for breakfast, BLTs for lunch, or pork chops for dinner. He believes that what was detestable for the Israelites, Jesus, and the disciples thousands of years ago is still filthy today.

Sitting outdoors in Aosta, I wasn't about to order *pizza con prosciutto* just because I was visiting the land where pizza was invented. So Nicole ordered vegetarian pizzas for us and tuna salads with *aceto balsamico* for the boys, figuring that those were safe bets.

Twenty minutes later, the pizzas arrived at our table with a flourish, which prompted chuckles from Nicole and me. Draped across our pizzas were generous slices of thin Parma ham and cut-up bits of hot dogs. *Some vegetarian pizza.*

Nicole politely explained to the waiter that we didn't want pizzas with ham. A quizzical look came over his face. The idea that *anyone* on the Italian boot turning up his or her nose at *pizza con prosciutto* didn't register. *Mamma mia, impossibilita!*

The waiter left the table mumbling something in Italian, no doubt cursing his luck that three Americans and a Swiss happened to sit down at his restaurant that afternoon. Then a few minutes later, he returned with Mike and Jordan's tuna salads, which were liberally topped with diced-up weenies!

They laughed it off and pushed the weenies aside while they picked their way through the salad. Twenty minutes later, two new pizzas, *senza prosciutto,* arrived at our table, but if you can believe this, they were topped with slices of hot dogs again! Since we were famished and didn't want to create an international incident, we removed the hot dogs and the cheese underneath them and ate what was left.

**Jordan:** Why did our table make such a big deal about eating pork? Because pork, along with rabbit, horsemeat (popular in Europe, if you can believe it), certain birds like eagles and vultures; bottom-feeders like shrimp, catfish, and eel; and hard-shelled crustaceans like crabs, clams, and lobster are all meats that God called detestable or "unclean" in the Old Testament.

I devoted several pages in *The Great Physician's Rx for Health and Wellness* to describing what God had to say about eating clean versus unclean animals. He spoke in rather direct terms to Moses when He declared, "Of all the animals that live on land, these are the ones you may eat: You may eat any animal that has a split hoof completely divided and that chews the cud" (Lev. 11:2–3, NIV). Well, that certainly culls the herd. Animals with split hooves that munch on green grass include cows, goats, sheep, oxen, deer, buffalo, and other wild game. Camels chew the cud, but they don't have split hooves, so they don't make the cut. Neither do badgers, rabbits, and pigs. "You must not eat their meat or touch their carcasses; they are unclean for you," the Lord said in verse 8 (NIV).

I know that pork is as all-American as Chevrolets, hot dogs, and apple pie, but when it comes to hot dogs, they are made from pork "products," including ground-up snouts and lips. Don't take my word for it. No less an authority than a U.S. Department of Agriculture official, quoted in *Hog Farm* magazine, confirmed that "hot dogs contain skeletal muscles, along with parts of pork stomach, snout, intestines, spleens, edible fat [which the Bible also calls detestable], and yes, lips." Don't forget the preservatives, to keep this disgusting ground-up mixture all "fresh," but I digress.[24]

Pork, marketed as the nation's "other white meat," is a staple of the American diet. It's not unusual for folks to eat pork three times a day: bacon or sausage in the morning, a ham sandwich at lunchtime, and pork chops and a salad with bacon bits for dinner. Fast food establishments have watched their earnings sizzle by topping every hamburger and chicken sandwich in sight with strips of salty bacon; they go by names like Big Bacon Classic, Big Country Bacon, Cravin' Bacon Cheeseburger, Mesquite Bacon Cheeseburger, and Arch Deluxe with Bacon. Pork is, in fact, the world's most widely eaten meat, despite being an abomination to Jews and Muslims around the globe.[25] This is what writer Stephan Jack had to say about pigs: "Pigs can eat nearly anything that remotely resembles food, including stuff that humans choose not to ingest or could not digest—picture the classic image of the slop bucket and you get the idea. They can even derive nutrition from human excrement, eliminating a sanitary problem for their human masters in the process.[26]

This quote illustrates the fundamental difference between pigs—which eat any swill, any pail of fecal matter thrown their way—and animals that take their time chewing grass and grains that rise out of the earth. As much as the National Pork Producers Council wants to put a positive spin on things, God wasn't fooling around when he labeled pigs as detestable or unclean animals. Scripture says, "A washed pig returns to the mud" (2 Peter 2:22 NLT). Since God created pigs, He understands their fast-acting physiology. Pigs come with a simple stomach arrangement: whatever gets eaten wends its way through the digestive tract very quickly, not allowing enough time for proper digestion of nutrients or the elimination of wastes. So a pig can chomp on a pail of you-know-what from the outhouse and not be bothered in the least. They will even eat their *own* excrement if hungry enough. (Remember, you are what they ate!)

**Nicki:** To finish the "Three Meals, Three Countries" story, we left Aosta with three shopping bags filled with various whole-grain breads, Greek-style yogurt, Italian honey, fruits of the region, and raw nuts. When we arrived back in Switzerland, we set the delicious foods on the dining room table of Nicole's chalet and served ourselves a "farmer's banquet" as we chuckled about those pork pizzas in Italy.

### *Ordering Off the Menu*
*by Nicki Rubin*

Maybe you're wondering, *But what about eating out?* Good question. How *do* you eat healthy in a restaurant?

Generally speaking, the higher up the "food chain" you go in the restaurant world, the better quality food you'll receive at your table. Restaurants seem to charge a premium for serving the freshest, healthiest food, but that's because grass-fed beef, free-range chicken, wild-caught fish, and organic produce are more expensive than boxed, frozen hamburger patties and cans of fruit cocktail in sweet syrup. Still, I don't think you have to empty your wallet to eat well.

When choosing restaurants, we gravitate toward those that serve fish. And I'm not talking about Red Lobster, which is known for its shrimp and lobster meals. I'm talking about wild-caught tuna or sockeye salmon with vegetables; you can't get any healthier than that. We've had excellent luck at Thai restaurants, as well as some Japanese eateries. Many of the new Asian-fusion restaurant chains, including P.F. Chang's, will even serve you brown rice (also healthy!) upon request.

## WHAT TO SHOP FOR, WHAT TO SERVE

**Jordan:** Many people ask me, "Jordan, what kinds of foods should I be buying? What are the best, most nutritious foods to serve?"

I've prepared a comprehensive list of foods in three categories, based on the acronym EAT:

- *E* stands for Extraordinary.
- *A* stands for Average.
- *T* stands for Trouble.

Obviously, you want to fill your shopping cart with foods from the Extraordinary category.

In the charts below, each category lists foods in descending order based on their health-giving qualities. Foods at the top of the list are healthier than those at the bottom. It's best to consume foods from the Extraordinary category between 50 and 75 percent of the time.

## EXTRAORDINARY FOODS

***Meat*** *(grass-fed organic is best)*

beef
buffalo
elk
goat
lamb
meat-bone soup or stock
veal
venison
beef or buffalo hot dogs (with no pork casing)
beef or buffalo sausage (with no pork casing)
jerky (with no chemicals, nitrates, or nitrites)
liver and heart (must be organic)

***Fish*** (*wild- or ocean-caught is best, and the fish must have fins and scales)*

cod
sardines (canned in water or olive oil only)
fish soup or stock
scrod
grouper
sea bass
haddock
snapper
halibut
sole
herring
tilapia
mahi-mahi
trout

orange roughy
pompano
salmon
tuna
wahoo
whitefish

***Poultry*** *(pastured and organic is best)*

chicken
duck
poultry-bone soup or stock
Cornish game hen
guinea fowl
turkey
chicken or turkey bacon (with no pork casing)
chicken or turkey hot dogs (with no pork casing)
chicken or turkey sausage (with no pork casing)

***Lunch Meat*** *(organic, free-range, and hormone-free is best)*

chicken
roast beef
turkey

***Eggs*** *(high omega-3/DHA or organic are best)*

caviar and salmon roe (must be fresh, not preserved, and must not come from the sturgeon, which is an unclean fish)
chicken eggs (whole with yolk)
duck eggs (whole with yolk)

***Dairy*** *(organic is best)*

goat's milk plain whole yogurt
homemade kefir made from raw cow's milk
homemade kefir made from raw goat's milk
organic cow's milk yogurt or kefir
raw cow's milk hard cheeses
raw cream
raw goat's milk hard cheeses

*Fats and Oils (organic is best)*

avocado
butter, cow's milk
butter, cow's milk, raw, grass fed (not for cooking)
butter, goat's milk
butter, goat's milk, raw (not for cooking)
coconut milk/cream (canned)
oil, butter (ghee)
oil, coconut, extra-virgin (best for cooking)
oil, expeller-pressed peanut
oil, expeller-pressed sesame
oil, olive, extra-virgin (not for cooking)
oil, unrefined flaxseed (not for cooking)
oil, unrefined hemp seed (not for cooking)

*Vegetables (organic fresh or frozen is best)*

asparagus
artichokes (French, not Jerusalem)
beets
broccoli
Brussels sprouts
cabbage
cauliflower
corn
carrots
celery
cucumbers
eggplant
garlic
lettuce (all kinds)
mushrooms
okra
onions
peas
peppers
pumpkins
spinach
string beans
sweet potatoes
tomatoes
white potatoes
squash (winter or summer)
leafy greens (kale, collards, broccoli rabe, mustard greens)
salad greens (radicchio, escarole, endive)

raw fermented veggies (no vinegar)
sea vegetables (kelp, dulse, nori, kombu, and hijiki)
sprouts (broccoli, sunflower, pea shoots, radish, etc.)

***Fruits** (organic fresh or frozen is best)*

apples
apricots
bananas
blackberries
blueberries
dates
figs
dried fruits (no sugar or sulfites)
grapefruit
grapes
kiwis
lemons
limes
mangos
melons
oranges
papayas
peaches
pears
pineapples
plums
prunes
raisins
raspberries
strawberries

***Grains and Starchy Carbohydrates** (organic is best, and whole grains and flours are best if soaked for six to twelve hours before cooking)*

amaranth
buckwheat
millet
quinoa
sprouted Essene bread
sprouted Ezekiel-type bread
sprouted whole-grain cereal
fermented whole-grain sourdough bread

***Sweeteners***

date sugar
unheated raw honey

***Beans and Legumes*** *(best if soaked for twelve hours)*

- black beans
- black-eyed peas
- broad beans
- garbanzo beans
- kidney beans
- lentils
- lima beans
- miso
- natto
- navy beans
- pinto beans
- red beans
- soybeans (edamame)
- split peas
- tempeh
- white beans

***Nuts and Seeds*** *(organic, raw, and/or soaked is best)*

- almonds (raw or dry roasted)
- almond butter (raw or roasted)
- Brazil nuts (raw)
- flaxseeds (raw and ground)
- hazelnuts (raw)
- hemp seed butter (raw)
- hemp seeds (raw)
- macadamia nuts (raw or dry roasted)
- pecans (raw or dry roasted)
- pumpkin seed butter (raw or roasted)
- pumpkin seeds (raw or dry roasted)
- sunflower butter (raw or roasted)
- sunflower seeds (raw or dry roasted)
- tahini (raw or roasted)
- walnuts (raw or dry roasted)

***Condiments, Spices, and Seasonings*** *(organic is best)*

- salsa (fresh or canned)
- apple cider vinegar
- Celtic Sea Salt
- guacamole (fresh)

Herbamare seasoning
herbs and spices (no added stabilizers)
ketchup (no sugar)
mustard
omega-3 mayonnaise
other marinades (no canola oil)
real salt
sea salt
soy sauce (wheat-free, tamari)
tomato sauce (no added sugar)
umeboshi paste
other salad dressings (no canola oil)
raw salad dressings and marinades
flavoring extracts, such as vanilla or almond (alcohol based, no sugar)

***Snacks***

healthy food bars
carob powder
flaxseed crackers
goat's milk protein powder
healthy macaroons
healthy trail mix
organic chocolate spreads
organic cocoa powder
raw food snacks

***Beverages***

coconut water
purified, nonchlorinated water
lacto-fermented beverages
raw vegetable or fruit juices
natural sparkling water, no carbonation added
unsweetened or honey-sweetened herbal teas

## AVERAGE FOODS

Foods in the average category should make up no more than 25 to 50 percent of your daily diet. If you are currently in poor health, consume these foods sparingly.

***Dairy*** *(organic is best)*

goat's milk
almond milk
amazake
cheese (cow, goat, or sheep)
cow's milk
cow's milk cottage cheese

cream cheese
cultured whole soy yogurt
fat-free yogurt
heavy cream
low-fat yogurt
oat milk
plain sour cream
rice milk
soy milk

***Fats and Oils***

safflower oil
soy oil
sunflower oil

***Vegetables*** *(organic is best)*

canned vegetables

***Fruits*** *(organic is best)*

canned fruit in its own juices

***Grains and Starchy Carbohydrates*** *(whole grains and whole-grain flours are healthiest if soaked for twelve hours before consuming)*

brown rice
barley
corn
kamut
oats
rye
spelt
wheat
white potatoes
whole-grain dried cereal
whole-grain pasta (wheat, kamut, or spelt)

***Sweeteners***

honey
agave nectar
barley malt
brown rice syrup
maple syrup
organic dehydrated cane juice
Stevia
xylitol

***Nuts, Seeds, Beans, and Legumes*** *(organic is best)*

cashews (raw or dry roasted) | peanuts (dry roasted)
peanut butter (roasted) | tofu
soynut butter (in small quantities)
cashew butter (raw or roasted, in small quantities)

***Condiments, Spices, and Seasonings*** *(organic chemical- and preservative-free is best)*

ketchup | marinade
mayonnaise | pickled ginger
salad dressing | wasabi

***Snacks***

healthy popcorn | baked corn or rice chips
rice protein | soy protein (nongenetically modified)
milk or whey protein powder from cow's milk

***Beverages*** *(organic is best)*

fresh ground coffee (limit to one cup per day)
pasteurized fruit juices (not from concentrate)
pasteurized vegetable juices

## TROUBLE FOODS

Foods in the trouble category should be consumed with extreme caution. You and your family should greatly limit these foods or avoid them completely.

***Meat***

pork | bacon
emu | ham
ostrich | imitation meat products (soy)
rabbit | sausage (pork)
veggie burgers

***Fish and Seafood***

All shellfish, including:

crabs
lobsters
oysters
shrimp
eel
squid (calamari)
clams
mussels
scallops
catfish
fried or breaded fish
shark

***Poultry***

fried or breaded chicken

***Lunch Meat***

corned beef
soy lunch meat
ham

***Eggs***

imitation eggs (e.g., Egg Beaters)

***Dairy***

American cheese (singles)
homogenized milk
processed cheese food
soy cheese
commercial ice cream with sugar
low-fat or skim milk
rice cheese
yogurt with sugar or artificial sweeteners
any dairy product with added stabilizers, preservatives, sugars, or artificial sweeteners

***Fats and Oils***

canola oil
corn oil
lard
shortening
any partially hydrogenated oil
cottonseed oil
margarine

*Fruits*

canned fruits in syrup

*Grains and Starchy Carbohydrates*

baked goods
dried cereal with sugar
instant oatmeal
pastries
white or unbleached flour
white rice
bread or crackers made with white or unbleached flour
pastas made with white or unbleached flour

*Sweeteners*

sugar
all artificial sweeteners, including:
acesulfame K
aspartame (Equal)
maltitol
sorbitol
sucralose (Splenda)
saccharin (Sweet'N Low, Sugar Twin)
corn syrup
high-fructose corn syrup

*Nuts and Seeds*

honey-roasted nuts
nuts roasted in oil

*Condiments, Spices, and Seasonings*

all spices that contain added sugar or preservatives

*Beverages*

commercial beer and wine
chlorinated tap water
fruit juices or drinks made from concentrate
fruit juices or drinks with artificial flavors
sodas

*Miscellaneous*

snack foods with sugar, partially hydrogenated oils, artificial sweeteners, or unbleached flour

*What Women Are Saying*
*by Meredith Berkich*

When my husband, Mike, and I got married, I was a college freshman modeling for department stores and clothing companies like Pendleton Woolen Mills. I was a size 2 petite who could eat absolutely everything without having anything stick to me. My husband—who was an outside linebacker for the University of Oregon and would later play a season of pro football before getting injured—made a friendly agreement with me that we would always maintain a hundred-pound difference between us. Physical appearance and conditioning were an incredibly important part of our lives.

That agreement happened twenty-four years and forty-five pounds ago. Mike maintained his athletic physique, but I became softer and wider as children were born and the years passed. I began to feel guilty because I wanted my husband to "rejoice in the bride of his youth," as the Bible says in Proverbs 5:18, and my lack of discipline was really showing in the mirror—not to mention in my closet.

I felt that my appearance was making it challenging for Mike to maintain a deep attraction and respect for me, which wasn't fair to either him or our marriage. To my husband's credit, he never once made me feel unattractive or unlovely.

It wasn't the guilt, however, that drove me to take drastic measures to regain control of my life; it was several events that occurred over the past year that resulted in the most stressful time period in my personal history. My grandmother was diagnosed with incurable cancer—the same disease had taken my mother several years before. The responsibility of being her sole health-care provider fell completely on my shoulders, and when she passed away, I was left with the responsibility of handling her estate.

At the same time, my husband and I decided to sell our business, our oldest child went off to college, and I started a new job as vice president of a start-up company. To help ease the added stress, I would head straight for the cupboards and the refrigerator the moment I walked in the door at night and start grazing. This type of behavior was totally out of character for me, but emotional eating provided comfort when life all around me was spinning out of control.

In the past, I had tried just about every diet out there. I ate nothing but cabbage soup for a week until my family banished the Crock-Pot from the house because the smell permeated every nook and cranny of our home. I went on the watermelon diet, the grapefruit diet, and the salad-dressing diet, where I added ginger to my salad because it supposedly burned calories. Some pounds came off, but they always came right back on.

When I heard about Jordan Rubin's new program, the Great Physician's Rx, I couldn't wait to get started. Jordan had taken the wisdom he acquired in a short period of time through his own personal health crisis and incorporated it into a program that addressed the health challenges in my own life. I needed to submit my life once again to the authority and guidance of a loving God, to give up earthly habits and trust the Holy Spirit to empower discipline where I would fail in my own strength.

It really struck me when Jordan said it wasn't enough to eat well if you're not addressing a plethora of issues: emotional and spiritual, hygiene and environmental, nutritional and physical. I embarked on the 49-day program with the confidence and attitude that "with God, all things are possible," and I let go and let God.

The weight that came off was fabulous—over twenty-five pounds, which isn't easy at forty-something. About halfway through the Great Physician's Rx's 49-day plan, I noticed I was sleeping better, and my energy returned. Peace was restored to my soul, and my confidence returned.

At the end of the program, Mike and I went shopping at a department store, where a salesgirl who has helped me pick out clothes for several years, said, "Wow!" when she took a look at me. "What size can I get for you now?"

With a song in my heart, I replied, "Esther, make that a size 6, please."

Thank you, Jordan. It's great to be *me* again!

## Rx THE GREAT PHYSICIAN'S Rx FOR WOMEN'S HEALTH: EAT TO LIVE

- *Feed yourself and your family foods that God created, in a form that is healthy for the body.*
- *If you're trying to lose weight, choose foods high in nutrients, healthy fats, and fiber, and stay away from low-carb and low-fat diets.*
- *To improve the appearance of your skin and maintain your ideal weight, drink a half ounce of water per pound of body weight daily, and more if you exercise.*
- *Practice partial fasting one day per week.*
- *Increase your consumption of raw fruits and vegetables a few days before and during your menstrual cycle.*
- *Consume cultured whole milk dairy products high in calcium, and green veggies high in magnesium for strong bones.*
- *Eat wild-caught fish liberally. These are high in omega-3 fatty acids.*

- *Don't drink diet soft drinks; choose water and fresh fruit and veggie juices instead.*

- *Avoid processed foods, including dessert items. Many contain hydrogenated oils and trans fats.*

## THE GREAT PHYSICIAN'S RX FOR WOMEN'S HEALTH WEEK #1

If you're ready to follow the Great Physician's Rx for health and wellness program, then I've prepared a 49-day plan that will revolutionize how you eat and live. This seven-week plan is designed to improve your health, help you lose weight, and lay a strong foundation for a lifetime of superb health for you and your family.

In the first week, you'll ease into the Great Physician's Rx 7 Weeks of Wellness health plan by eating what you normally would for a few meals, but it won't be long before you're eating to live at *every* meal. Yes, this menu plan will involve some changes in your shopping habits, but you will notice a big difference in the way you feel.

The following listed meals and snacks are merely suggestions. Please feel free to adapt the 49-day meal plan to fit your needs, but make sure to consume Extraordinary foods most of the time and Average foods the rest of the time. (Refer back to the EAT list earlier in this chapter.)

This chapter only includes the first week of the 49-day plan. Subsequent weeks will be found within the remaining six Keys. Each day's eating and supplement plan aims to provide you with the following:

- three meals and up to two snacks per day
- between 1,500 and 1,800 nutrient-dense calories
- between 60 and 90 grams of high-quality protein
- a minimum of seven servings of fruits and veggies per day

- 35 to 50 grams of fiber per day
- more than 1,500 mg of calcium per day
- eight to twelve 8-ounce glasses of water per day

Finally, I urge you to visit www.BiblicalHealthInstitute.com and click on the GPRx Resource Guide to learn more about the specific food brands and nutritional supplements I recommend.

### Need Recipes?

*For a detailed list of more than 250 healthy and delicious recipes, including those contained in the Great Physician's Rx 49-day health plan, please visit www.BiblicalHealthInstitute.com.*

### Day 1

***Breakfast***

Eat what you consider to be your normal breakfast.

***Lunch***

Eat what you consider to be your normal lunch.

***Dinner***

grilled chicken

baked sweet potato with butter

green salad with red or yellow peppers, red onions, green or red cabbage, celery, cucumbers, and carrots

healthy salad dressing with olive oil and/or high-lignan flaxseed oil

***Snack/Dessert***

Eat what you consider to be your normal snack or dessert.

## DAY 2

***Breakfast***

Eat what you consider to be your normal breakfast.

***Lunch***

Eat what you consider to be your normal lunch.

***Dinner***

broiled or baked fish of your choice

brown rice

green salad with red or yellow peppers, red onions, green or red cabbage, celery, cucumbers, and carrots

healthy salad dressing with olive oil and/or high-lignan flaxseed oil

***Snack/Dessert***

whole food meal replacement powder (with beta-glucans from soluble oat fiber) mixed in 12 ounces of water

one piece of fruit and 1 ounce of cheese

## DAY 3

*You will notice that some items in the meal plans that follow are italicized. You can find the recipes for these—and over other 250 delicious and healthy recipes—at www.BiblicalHealthInstitute.com.*

*Breakfast*

Eat what you consider to be your normal breakfast.

*Lunch*

green salad with 3 ounces of tuna (low-mercury, high omega-3) and carrots, red onions, cucumbers, and yellow peppers

salad dressing with one tablespoon of extra-virgin olive oil or high-lignan flaxseed oil

one piece of fruit

*Dinner*

*Herb-Baked Salmon with Creamed-Style Spinach*

quinoa with onions, peas, and carrots

green salad with red or yellow peppers, red onions, green or red cabbage, celery, cucumbers, and carrots

healthy salad dressing with olive oil and/or high-lignan flaxseed oil

*Snack/Dessert*

apple cinnamon whole food bar (with beta-glucans from soluble oat fiber)

apple with almond or sesame butter (tahini)

## DAY 4

*You will notice that some items in the meal plans that follow are italicized. You can find the recipes for these—and over other 250 delicious and healthy recipes—at www.BiblicalHealthInstitute.com.*

*Breakfast*

two eggs (omega-3 or organic, and prepared as desired)

sprouted toast with butter

grapefruit

***Lunch***

low-mercury, high omega-3 tuna on sprouted or yeast-free whole-grain bread with lettuce, tomato, and sprouts

one piece of fruit

***Dinner***

*Chicken Piccata*

*Millet Corn Casserole*

*Garlicky Green Beans*

***Snack/Dessert***

whole food meal replacement powder (with beta-glucans from soluble oat fiber) mixed in 12 ounces of water

raw veggies and hummus, salsa, or guacamole

### DAY 5 (PARTIAL-FAST DAY)

*You will notice that some items in the meal plans that follow are italicized. You can find the recipes for these—and over other 250 delicious and healthy recipes—at www.BiblicalHealthInstitute.com.*

***Upon Waking***

Drink 12 to 16 ounces of water.

***Breakfast***

none (partial-fast day)

Drink 12 ounces of water.

***Between Breakfast and Lunch***

Drink 12 ounces of water.

*Lunch*

none (partial-fast day)

Drink 12 ounces of water.

*Between Lunch and Dinner*

Drink 12 ounces of water.

*Dinner*

During dinner, drink 8 ounces of water.

*Chicken Soup*

fermented veggies

green salad with red or yellow peppers, red onions, green or red cabbage, celery, cucumbers, and carrots

healthy salad dressing with olive oil and/or high-lignan flaxseed oil

*Snacks*

none (partial-day fast)

## DAY 6

*You will notice that some items in the meal plans that follow are italicized. You can find the recipes for these—and over other 250 delicious and healthy recipes—at www.BiblicalHealthInstitute.com.*

*Upon Waking*

Drink 12 to 16 ounces of water.

*Breakfast*

During breakfast, drink 8 ounces of water.

For a healthy smoothie, mix the following in a blender:

8 ounces plain whole milk, yogurt, or kefir

1 tablespoon honey

1/2 cup fresh or frozen fruit (bananas, peaches, berries, pineapple, etc.)

1 teaspoon high-lignan flaxseed oil

1 serving of protein powder (optional)

***Between Breakfast and Lunch***

Drink 8 ounces of water.

***Lunch***

During lunch, drink 8 ounces of water.

green salad with 3 ounces of salmon and carrots, red onions, cucumbers, and yellow peppers

healthy salad dressing with one tablespoon of extra-virgin olive oil or high-lignan flaxseed oil

one piece of fruit

***Between Lunch and Dinner***

Drink 12 ounces of water.

***Dinner***

During dinner, drink 8 ounces of water.

*Filet of Grass-Fed Beef*

*Mushroom Soup*

steamed asparagus with butter

green salad with red or yellow peppers, red onions, green or red cabbage, celery, cucumbers, and carrots

healthy salad dressing with olive oil and/or high-lignan flaxseed oil

***Snack/Dessert***

green superfood whole food bar (with beta-glucans from soluble oat fiber)

raw nuts, seeds, and dried fruit

## DAY 7

*You will notice that some items in the meal plans that follow are italicized. You can find the recipes for these—and over other 250 delicious and healthy recipes—at www.BiblicalHealthInstitute.com.*

***Upon Waking***

Drink 12 to 16 ounces of water.

***Breakfast***

During breakfast, drink 8 ounces of water.

1/2 cup organic cottage cheese

fruit (berries, peaches, or pineapple, etc.)

1 teaspoon raw honey

1/2 teaspoon high-lignan flaxseed oil (optional)

hot tea with honey

***Between Breakfast and Lunch***

Drink 12 ounces of water.

***Lunch***

During lunch, drink 8 ounces of water.

turkey on sprouted or yeast-free whole-grain bread with lettuce, tomato, and sprouts

one piece of fruit

***Between Lunch and Dinner***

Drink 12 ounces of water.

***Dinner***

During dinner, drink 8 ounces of water.

*Tropical Chicken and Vegetable Kabobs*

brown rice

steamed vegetable medley

*Snack/Dessert*

whole food meal replacement powder (with beta-glucans from soluble oat fiber) mixed in 12 ounces of water

*Blueberry* or *Peach Cobbler*

# Key #2

## *Supplement Your Diet with Whole Food Nutritionals, Living Nutrients, and Superfoods*

**Nicki:** A week or two after our first date, Jordan asked me to join him for the wedding of one his best friends, where he dressed up since he was one of the groomsmen. At the reception, the DJ revved up the wedding party with a string of '80s hits. After working the dance floor to a fever pitch, the swinging disc jockey played a slow song. Jordan took my hand in his and wrapped his arm gingerly around my waist. I drew close to him—and was immediately assaulted by the rankest smell. His body *reeked* of garlic!

The pungent odor nearly knocked me out. Nobody stinks this bad! Jordan smelled like someone had given him a deep-body massage with fresh garlic cloves . . . but I kept that to myself.

A few days later, he dropped by my apartment after work. Again, garlic odor trailed him as if he were Pepé Le Pew. Sooner or later I had to say something, so I worked up my courage and casually asked him, "Hey, what's going on with the garlic thing? Every time I'm around you, I smell garlic on you."

Jordan wasn't embarrassed at all. "Garlic? Oh yeah. I'm doing this juice fast, and I'm adding the juice of nine cloves of raw garlic to the mix. You can really tell?"

"Can I tell?!! Are you kidding me?"

Jordan, I soon discovered, was always trying out some new nutritional strategy he heard about. He was fascinated by nutrition and health, which explains why he wasn't afraid to get up close and personal with raw garlic.

**Jordan:** My garlic story is good for a laugh today, but if I can turn serious for a moment, I believe it's crucial to enhance our diets with the *right* supplements to ensure an adequate supply of essential nutrients to maintain good health. Supplements help protect us against toxins and prevent cell damage. They are used to fight disease and combat early aging. Supplements such as vitamin C and E are known for their protective functions against the impact of toxins. They also help the body detoxify.[1]

"Research has shown that each part of the body contains high concentrations of certain nutrients," wrote Phyllis Balch, author of *Prescription for Nutritional Healing*. "A deficiency of these nutrients will cause the body part to malfunction and eventually break down—and, like dominoes—other body parts will follow. To keep this from happening, we need a proper diet and appropriate nutritional supplements. If we do not give ourselves the proper nutrients, we can impair the body's normal functions and cause ourselves great harm."[2]

Many people understand that nutritional supplements are an integral part of good health. While more than 70 percent of us swallow multivitamins and other vitamins and minerals regularly,[3] the problem is that many of the supplements found in retail outlets are made from isolated or synthetic nutrients that are not in the same form as the nutrients found in healthy foods.

Just as the nation's bakeries have found a way to make bread cheaper through using "enriched" white flour, nutritional companies have learned how to produce cheaper supplements by synthetically creating complex structures like vitamin E, vitamin C, and vitamin A. Their research and development teams work to discover how to synthesize compounds that *appear* to be the same as the nutrients that God created in foods, but they aren't utilized by the body as food. It's like the difference between raw honey and white sugar, or brown rice and white rice: the former is nutritious; the latter is refined and missing vital nutrients.

I'm convinced that the most effective supplements—known as "whole food" supplements—are derived from foods that God created, not chemicals created in a lab. Whole food supplements are dried extracts from whole food complexes. Their nutrients are produced by probiotic fermentation, which means that the nutrient complexes are put through a fermentation process similar to the body's digestive process. Thus, the isolated nutrients are recombined in the same form found in food so the body can recognize and utilize them better. The reasons we should take supplements are compelling:

1. The fruits and vegetables coming from our farm fields don't contain as many enzymes, minerals, and healthy microorganisms as they did in generations past.
2. The typical American diet, with its glamorous array of technofoods, replete with empty calories and refined carbohydrates, strays far from God's design.

Supplements can help bridge that nutritional gap, though dietary supplements are just what they say they are—*supplements*, not a *substitute* for an inadequate diet. You can't feast on junk food and expect a bottle of pills to save you. That said, I believe supplements make nutritional sense for women. High-quality whole food nutritionals and superfoods can help boost your immune system; reduce risk factors of osteoporosis, breast cancer, diabetes, and heart disease; and ensure healthy skin, hair, and nails. Pregnant women profit from supplements because they need more folic acid, iron, and other nutrients. Menopausal women battling osteoporosis need extra minerals to replace those lost through bone depletion. Mineral deficiencies can lead to vague symptoms of fatigue and poor concentration. Supplements can help reverse these conditions.[4]

Many women are aware that nutritional deficiencies are a major reason why they go through the day lacking vitality. Research shows that women are more likely than men to take supplements, and usage increases with age. For instance, 35 percent of women ages eighteen to forty-four use vitamin or mineral supplements (as compared to 24 percent of men). The number increases to 51 percent for women ages forty-five to sixty-four, and 59 percent for women sixty-five and older,[5] probably because of osteoporosis concerns.

In a nutshell, the foundational nutritional supplements you want to add to your daily regimen are whole food multivitamins, omega-3 cod-liver oil, whole food calcium, a magnesium formula, and a cleansing green food fiber blend with flaxseed. Since moms are usually the family's "health coach," I encourage you—if you are a mother—to get the entire family on board. The following supplements are a good place to start.

### *A Primer on Vitamins and Minerals*

Vitamins and minerals help regulate metabolism; assist the biochemical processes that release energy from digested foods; and support the formation of hormones, blood cells, nervous system chemicals, and genetic material.[6] At the same time, there are some key differences between vitamins and minerals:

- *Vitamins*, which are essential for life, are organic substances that the body cannot make. (Exceptions are vitamin D and niacin.) Every single organ in the body needs vitamins to perform its functions; otherwise, we will perish. Vitamins fall into two main groups. Some are *water-soluble*, which means that water is required for their absorption and that they are excreted in urine. There are at least nine different water-soluble vitamins, including vitamin C and the eight different B vitamins. The other vitamins are *fat-soluble*, which require a certain amount of fat to be absorbed and stored in the body. The four main fat-soluble vitamins are A, D, K, and E.
- *Minerals* are inorganic substances that are also vital to the body. Calcium, magnesium, iron, phosphorus, potassium, sodium, and sulfur are *macrominerals*. Zinc and chromium are considered to be *trace minerals*, required in relatively small amounts. Minerals are necessary for the proper functioning of vitamins, enzymes, hormones, and other metabolic activities within the body, but they are not easily absorbed.

## Whole Food Multivitamins

For many years, conventional medicine stated that nutritional supplements weren't necessary if you ate a healthy, wholesome diet. Some physicians said you were throwing money down the toilet, and all you had to show for it was glow-in-the-dark urine.

James F. Balch, MD, and Mark Stengler, ND, summed up the prevailing attitude in their book, *Prescription for Natural Cures,* while noting that traditional medicine is coming to realize that nutritional supplements can be a key component in the prevention and treatment of many health conditions:

> To the detriment of the public, most conventional doctors in the past have had little support for the use of these nontoxic nutrients [referring to nutritional supplements]. Fortunately, times are changing. Two decades ago, the prestigious *Journal of the American Medical Association (JAMA)* advised that there was no evidence that healthy people would benefit from taking multivitamins. In June 2002, *JAMA* published an article that was a complete turnaround on the use of nutritional supplements. The authors of this study concluded that vitamin deficiency was an apparent cause of chronic diseases. Considering that only 20 percent of the population consumes the recommended minimum servings of fruits and vegetables each day, nutritional deficiencies are undoubtedly a widespread problem.[7]

I looked up the updated report from the *Journal of the American Medical Association,* and sure enough, it stated, "We recommend that all adults take a multivitamin daily."[8] I would amend that advice with the addition of two words: *whole food.*

Again, whole food multivitamins are made from concentrated whole foods and whole food compounds. Vitamins in whole food form have not been synthetically produced or "isolated" by white-coated researchers. Daniel H. Chong, ND, writing on the Web site of my friend, osteopathic physician

Joseph Mercola (www.mercola.com), used the analogy of an automobile to describe the difference between whole food supplements and those made from synthetic sources.

An automobile, Chong said, comes off an assembly line a wonderfully designed yet complex machine that needs all of its parts, in proper working condition, in order to run. You could never "isolate" the wheels, for instance, because your automobile wouldn't function like a car if it were up on blocks. Automobiles need every working part, from an engine to a steering wheel to turn signals, to operate the way it was designed to.

Multivitamin manufacturers who use isolated or "synthetic" vitamins and minerals are like those who scavenge through a junkyard, picking out parts they need to assemble an entire automobile, and throwing them together as best they can with the expectation of driving off to their next destination.[9]

I recommend you switch from the "one-a-day" multi you're using to a whole food multivitamin/mineral formulation. I've prepared a listing of my favorite brands of whole food multivitamins (as well as the other supplements discussed in this chapter) in the comprehensive GPRx Resource Guide at www.BiblicalHealthInstitute.com.

## OMEGA-3 COD-LIVER OIL

**Nicki:** When I was pregnant, Jordan told me that expectant moms who took omega-3 cod-liver oil during pregnancy and gave omega-3 cod-liver oil to their child during the first year of life were more likely to have children with higher IQs.[10] And so you can be sure that Joshua received tiny teaspoons of cod-liver oil before his first birthday.

Whenever Jordan speaks in churches or at health lectures, he sings the praises of omega-3 cod-liver oil, calling it his favorite supplement. He informs audiences that if they each took omega-3 cod-liver oil daily, they could greatly reduce the risk of many major illnesses; improve their immune systems and mood; and have stronger bones and healthier skin, hair, and nails. Study after study shows that omega-3 cod-liver oil is important for the development of the brain and nervous system, and that the rods and the cone of the eye's retina respond well to the nutrients contained in omega-3 cod-liver oil.

When Jordan extolled omega-3 cod-liver oil during our courtship, I read some of these studies for myself and wanted to take omega-3 cod-liver oil too, but I worried about the fishy smell and aftertaste. Fortunately, Jordan has formulated his own lemon-mint–flavored omega-3 cod-liver oil in liquid form; for the less brave, there is a capsule. During my pregnancy, I faithfully took one to three teaspoons of omega-3 cod-liver oil daily.

These days, Jordan and I are convinced that our two-year-old son, Joshua, is the Smartest Kid in the Whole Wide World, although I had to get after him for misspelling a few words on his latest research paper in pre-preschool. I'm kidding, of course, but I'm serious about how important omega-3 cod-liver oil is to my son's development as well as my continued good health. David Horrobin, an Oxford-educated medical doctor with a doctorate in neuroscience, who devoted much of his life to researching essential fatty acids, firmly believed that if parents want to prevent learning disabilities in their children, they should make sure to feed their sons and daughters a teaspoon or two of cod-liver oil daily.

In preparation for this chapter, I looked up the kids-are-smarter-when-Mom-takes-omega-3 cod-liver study online, which was initially reported in *Pediatrics* magazine in January 2003. I wanted to know if my memory was correct, and it was. Researchers in Oslo, Norway, once conducted a study of three hundred pregnant women over a five-year period. Half the women were given omega-3 cod-liver oil supplements, and the other half took corn oil supplements from their eighteenth week of pregnancy until three months after childbirth. When the offspring—eighty-four kids in all—reached four years of age, researchers conducted various assessments of intelligence. Those whose mothers received the omega-3 cod-liver oil scored higher on cognitive tests, or the equivalent of about four IQ points. All I can say is that Joshua better nail those SAT tests in about fifteen years!

*If You're Expecting or Nursing . . .*
*by Pancheta Wilson, MD*

If you are pregnant or nursing, you should consult with a doctor, a certified nutritionist, or a registered dietician before embarking on any type of supplement program. The nutritional value of a pregnant women's diet is just as important as the total caloric intake. During pregnancy, a woman's protein requirement is somewhat greater than normal. Talk to your doctor or nutritionist about taking iron, calcium, folate, and vitamin D supplements.

**Jordan:** The reason omega-3 cod-liver oil is such an outstanding supplement is that it contains four important nutrients that most of us are deficient in, including docosahexaenoic acid, or DHA, a type of omega-3 fatty acid. (Another excellent long-chain polyunsaturated omega-3 fat, eicosapentaenoic acid, or EPA, is also present in cod-liver oil.) Norwegian researchers theorize that DHA appears to have a positive effect in developing children.

I urge all women to add omega-3 cod-liver oil to their daily regimen.

**Nicki:** It's also important for children to take this supplement. We feed our son omega-3 cod-liver oil by putting a teaspoon in a special formula that Jordan created especially for him. (We'll share this formula in Jordan's upcoming book, *The Great Physician's Rx for Children's Health,* due out in January 2008.) I remind myself that my son is getting smarter with each teaspoon. Yet I know some moms may be wondering, *Why can't I just feed the kids fish instead of making them drink omega-3 cod-liver oil?*

**Jordan:** Eating fish is a good idea, but most kids don't like the oily taste of fatty fish like salmon, which are high in omega-3. But even if kids are served fatty fish a few times per week, they may still be missing out on the other two important nutrients found in omega-3 cod-liver oil—vitamins A and D.

Cod-liver oil contains more vitamins A and D per unit weight than any other common food, and these essential nutrients are difficult to obtain in the modern diet. Vitamin A is an important nutrient for the eyes and immune system because of how it impacts the integrity of the mucosal linings of the body, such as the gastrointestinal tract and the lungs. When a flu bug or a cold gets you down, the body "collects" all the vitamin A at hand to fight back the invaders. This is just one more reason to be sipping teaspoons of cod-liver oil during the cold and flu season.

Vitamin D is actually not a vitamin but a critical hormone the body requires to regulate the health of thirty different tissues and organs. The vitamin D in cod-liver oil helps build strong bones in children as they grow up, and at the other end of life's spectrum, it helps prevent osteoporosis in adults. Richard Hobday, PhD, author of *The Healing Sun*, points out that women begin to lose about 1 percent of their bone mass each year, starting between the ages of thirty and thirty-five. Bone loss accelerates after menopause since estrogen levels decline; we've all seen the sad image of a woman hunched over with a dowager's hump. In a review of women with osteoporosis that were hospitalized for hip fractures, 50 percent were found to have signs of vitamin D deficiency, according to the National Institutes of Health.[11]

Dr. Hobday says that the orthodox view is that osteoporosis is largely irreversible, so treatment is aimed at preventing further bone loss rather than rebuilding the remaining skeleton.[12] That's not his view, nor mine, because we are both convinced that the vitamin D in cod-liver oil is one of the most important supplements a women can take.

There is growing evidence that vitamin D helps protect against colorectal, breast, and ovarian cancers. Researcher Cedric Garland, a doctor of public health at the University of California at San Diego, has been studying the impact of vitamin D on cancer since the 1980s. Dr. Garland says the evidence of more than one thousand studies examining vitamin D and cancer suggests that a vitamin D deficiency is responsible for several thousand premature deaths each year from colon, breast, and ovarian cancer.[13]

William B. Grant, PhD, who has authored or coauthored more than sixty articles in peer-reviewed journals on the relationship between vitamin D and certain cancer risks, said that while a proper diet and exercise can reduce the risk of breast cancer, an additional way to lessen the threat is to get plenty of vitamin D. "Breast cancer risk could be cut in half by sufficient vitamin D levels," he wrote on the Sunlight, Nutrition, and Health Research Center (SUNARC) Web site that he founded.[14]

Although cod-liver oil hasn't gotten the respect it deserves over the years, I think that view is changing as more women hear about how helpful this nutritional supplement is to long-term health. I urge you to give cod-liver oil a try for a month. The Weston A. Price Foundation, founded upon the principles of nutrition pioneer Weston Price, called cod-liver oil the "number one superfood" and a "must" for women, especially those who are pregnant.

## PROBIOTICS

One of the main weapons that physicians and pediatricians employ is prescription antibiotics, which kill harmful bacteria that have invaded the body. Since their discovery in the 1930s, antibiotics have cured millions worldwide suffering from pneumonia, tuberculosis, and meningitis.

Consequently, many parents believe that bacteria are *bad* for you. In fact, I would wager that every time people hear the word *bacteria* on a TV ad, the adjective *harmful* has been placed in front of it. One popular mouthwash says their product "kills harmful bacteria on contact."

Yet some kinds of bacteria are not only good for the body but are *essential* to good health. Without the growth of beneficial bacteria in the digestive tract, the body would cease to function properly. When I was diagnosed with Crohn's disease, along with a host of other gastrointestinal and immune system ailments, I wasn't aware that the normal gastrointestinal tract contains hundreds of different species of *harmless* or even beneficial microorganisms, otherwise known as intestinal flora. *Probiotics*, which are living, direct-fed microbials (DFMs), promote the growth of beneficial bacteria in the intestines.

I believe some of the most important microorganisms that the body should receive are probiotic or "friendly" yeasts, such as *Saccharomyces boulardii* and soil-based organisms (SBOs) from the *Bacillus* family. Probiotic yeasts and SBOs are room-temperature stable, which means they do not require refrigeration, as most American-made probiotics do. They are not destroyed by most antibiotics, so they can be used during antibiotic therapy.

Probiotic yeasts have been shown to promote immune system health, digestion, and elimination, and SBOs are shown to have strong antimicrobial effects. Very few nutritional supplement companies in the United States are utilizing these effective probiotic organisms, but they can be found at companies listed in the GPRx Resource Guide at www.BiblicalHealthInstitute.com.

*The Issue of Estrogen Dominance*
*by Pancheta Wilson, MD*

Chances are, you've never heard of "estrogen dominance," a term coined by John Lee, MD, upon the release of his book *What Your Doctor May Not Tell You About Menopause: The Breakthrough Book on Natural Progesterone.*

Estrogen dominance occurs in women when there's an imbalance of estrogen and progesterone. Estrogen, a powerful steroid compound that functions as the primary female sex hormone, "dominates" the body up to the day ovulation occurs in the menstrual cycle, which is usually day 14. Then progesterone takes the lead as the body's dominant hormone until menstruation begins, which is usually day 28.

But for a certain number of women, follicles in the ovaries release too much estrogen during the first part of the menstrual cycle, causing a hormonal imbalance that may set off a wide range of physical ailments, including colon dysfunction, endometriosis, chronic candida overgrowth, allergies, lupus, fibroids, headaches, insomnia, mood swings, and bloating.

Dr. Lee says that a woman's hormonal balance begins to shift when she reaches her midthirties to late forties, the so-called *perimenopausal* years. The follicles' ability to mature an egg and release it sputters like a car engine trying to start on a cold morning. "During this time, the ovaries continue to produce estrogen sufficient for regular or irregular shedding, creating what I term 'estrogen dominance,'" wrote Dr. Lee.[15]

Dr. Lee recommends that women use natural progesterone cream to eliminate premenopausal symptoms and balance your hormones, as well as taking additional vitamins, minerals, fiber, and probiotics. I agree.

## GREEN FOODS

**Nicki:** Jordan and I had a different dating relationship. We didn't go out to eat like most courting couples do because he was trying to eat as perfectly as possible—all organic, all the time, remember? A romantic restaurant with muted lighting, a crisp white tablecloth, a stem rose in a vase, a scented candle, and limited "healthy" options on the menu would have to wait. It had only been a year since he had been horribly sick, so Jordan was still on the comeback trail.

A couple of months after the garlic episode, Jordan came by one evening, carrying a small box.

"What's that?"

"A mini blender and a bottle of a green food/fiber blend," Jordan responded. "I thought I'd make us a green drink." Jordan poured a few ounces of juice and water into the blender and mixed in the greenish brown powder.

"Try it." Jordan handed me my first organic "green drink," which was as dark green as a freshly mowed lawn of Kentucky bluegrass.

I took a small sip. It certainly didn't taste like a smoothie, and, *hmmm . . .* I could definitely taste the flavor of . . . grass clippings.

Jordan read my mind. "I've been experimenting with some different powders," he explained. "This one contains the dried fermented juice concentrates of wheat grass, oat grass, alfalfa grass, and barley grass." At the time, Jordan was working in a small nutritional supplement business, writing educational materials, taking phone orders, and formulating new products. Jordan's eyes lit up when he talked about the formulation process, which involved researching and developing what he called "whole food nutritional supplements." Testing was an important part of the R & D process, which explained his close-up episode with garlic.

I kept drinking Jordan's jade-colored drink, and I did get used to the "green" taste. What's more, I was actually drinking something very healthy for my body.

**Jordan:** Too many people, like the Nicki I knew before we married, never get around to eating leafy green vegetables, which are loaded with nutrients, including antioxidants, minerals, folate, and pigments such as chlorophyll, which work to prevent unstable molecules called free radicals from damaging healthy cells. Melissa Diane Smith, nutritionist and author of *Going Against the Grain: How Reducing and Avoiding Grains Can Revitalize Your Health*, said that most Americans don't even come close to the recent revised dietary recommendations of five to nine servings of fruits and vegetables a day.[16] As someone who pays attention to what people eat when I'm in a social setting, I heartily concur. Folks reach for chips and ranch dressing loaded with unhealthy fats—not broccoli sprigs or celery sticks—when they graze a buffet table. They fill up on the meat and potatoes, not the kale or collards.

Green foods, also known as "green superfoods," are a category of phytonutrient-rich nutritional supplements derived from green vegetables, cereal grasses, and microalgae. Leafy greens in dried form also contain as much calcium as milk.[17] Green foods are nutritionally vital to women because they are natural sources of vitamins, minerals, amino acids, enzymes, plant sterols, and other nutritional constituents. Look at the label of an excellent green food, and you'll see ingredients such as alfalfa, barley grass, wheat grass, chlorella, and spirulina.

The chlorophyll pigment in leafy green vegetables has been intensely researched for its benefits. Chlorophyll's chemical makeup strongly resembles hemoglobin, the portion of the blood that carries oxygen. When women don't have enough iron in their blood, their hemoglobin count drops, which means they're anemic. Green foods can bring that number up.

Research suggests that chlorophyll can be converted to hemoglobin, which builds iron levels and increases the flow of oxygen to all parts of the body.

Green foods also contain enzymes in addition to chlorophyll, which together help cleanse the body of accumulated toxins. During menstruation, when the uterus sheds its lining, green foods are especially helpful in replenishing nutrients to blood cells, fluids, and mucus. Since many women need to cleanse their bodies of toxins and keep their blood oxygen levels up—but fail to eat their five to nine servings of green vegetables and fruits daily—I recommend using a green food/fiber supplement.

**Nicki:** Although I turned up my nose the first few times Jordan whipped up green drinks for me, now it's one of my favorite supplements, especially when mixed with vegetable juice. One thing people notice within the first few days of taking a green superfood is that their elimination greatly improves. For many who suffer from occasional constipation, that will be a thing of the past.

I like to take green drinks in the morning and evening, either twenty minutes before dinner—which really helps me not to overeat—or after dinner before bed.

## Whole Food Fiber Supplements

**Jordan:** If you're eating five servings of leafy green vegetables per day, three pieces of raw fruits, three servings of sprouted grains, one whole avocado, one cup of soaked and cooked beans and legumes, several ounces of raw coconut, and about a half pound of raw nuts and seeds, then you don't have to worry about getting enough fiber. But I don't think you can find a single person in the United States faithfully following that diet.

Although we all fall short of the fiber we need to eat for good health, it's something we must pay attention to. Fiber is important because it keeps you regular, which is important to women. When I speak about how I overcame horrible digestive problems—from painful cramps to diarrhea to incessant heartburn—caused by Crohn's disease, I'm often swamped by women who approach me afterward about their digestive troubles. Many describe episodes of terrible abdominal cramps, dreadful bloating, recurring constipation, and knifelike jabs in the gut—the classic symptoms of irritable bowel syndrome (IBS), which is not a disease but a painful, life-altering functional digestive disorder in which the muscular contractions of the digestive tract become irregular and uncoordinated.

Of the 30 million Americans—10 percent of the U.S. population—plagued by some form of bowel distress, women outnumber men by a two-to-one margin. They suffer in silence for two reasons: (1) they are unaware of the true impact of the disorder, and (2) they aren't sure what they can do to improve their condition. Most women, even if they don't suffer from IBS, have experienced some digestive upsets, including postmeal bloating and occasional constipation. (I've written a book especially for those suffering from irritable bowel syndrome called *The Great Physician's Rx for Irritable Bowel Syndrome.* Check it out if constipation, diarrhea, or irritable bowel problems have taken over your life.)

Eating fiber-rich foods can set women down the path of regularity. Here's why: Fiber is the indigestible remnants of plant cells found in vegetables, fruits, whole grains, nuts, seeds, and beans. Fiber-rich foods take longer to break down and are partially indigestible, which means that as these foods work their way through the digestive tract, they absorb water and increase the elimination of fecal waste in the large intestine.

Good sources of fiber are berries, fruits with edible skins (apples, pears, and grapes), citrus fruits, whole non-gluten grains (quinoa, millet, amaranth, and buckwheat), green peas, carrots, cucumbers, zucchini, and tomatoes. Green leafy vegetables, such as romaine lettuce and spinach, are also fiber-rich. Eating foods high in fiber and low in starches will immediately improve your digestion and can lower blood cholesterol and triglycerides, but as I mentioned earlier, it's practically impossible to eat enough fiber these days.

A whole food fiber supplement can supply your body with the dietary fiber it needs to keep things moving. I believe the best fiber supplement for women is one that contains large amounts of flaxseeds and beta glucans from soluble oat bran fiber. Those two ingredients are excellent for promoting breast health, hormonal health, and blood sugar. Dietary fiber is best taken in a powder form in combination with a green superfood.

You can find out more about a fiber/green food combination that is excellent for everyday use in the GPRx Resource Guide at www.BiblicalHealthInstitute.com.

## *Flaxseed and Breast Health*
*by Jordan Rubin*

Flaxseeds are another fiber source that should be of interest to women. Ground organic flaxseeds are brimming with alpha-linolenic acid, an omega-3 fatty acid, as well as linolenic acid, an omega-6 fatty acid, which are known as "essential fatty acids," or EFAs. The body needs EFAs to manufacture and repair cell membranes, enabling the cells to expel harmful waste products and regulate body functions such as heart rate, blood pressure, fertility, and conception.

Dietary essential fatty acids common to flaxseed oil are ultimately converted to hormonelike substances known as *prostaglandins,* said Jade Beutler, coauthor of *Understanding Fats and Oils: Your Guide to Healing with Essential Fatty Acids.*[18] These prostaglandins regulate a host of bodily functions, including water retention, blood-clotting ability, nerve transmission, and inflammation and swelling.

The hulls of flaxseeds contain lignans, which are rich in phytoestrogens (estrogenlike substances from plants) and reduce excess estrogen from binding to receptor sites in breast tissue. This is important because a lifetime of exposure to estrogen is a well-known risk factor for contracting breast cancer. In a healthy body, cells divide at a controlled rate in order to grow and repair damaged tissues and replace dying cells. The body quickly recognizes any abnormal cells and removes them before they can cause harm. Cells are constantly dividing and growing; these around-the-clock activities keep us in good health. But when the body cannot check the growth of abnormal cells, these "bad" cells keep multiplying until a mass of tissue, called a growth or tumor, slowly emerges.[19]

When lignans are ingested, however, they work harmoniously with estrogen and estrogen receptors to bring the body back into balance, and to deal with any excessive or "bad" forms of estrogen that may adversely affect breast health. (Left unchecked, estrogen could result in rapid multiplication of breast cells, which can lead to the growth of tumors.)

Though it's more difficult to consume lignans because of our culture's preference for refined and processed shelf-stable foods, flaxseed is available in meal and seed form and as a key ingredient in the whole food fiber blend that I recommend women use daily. You can also find high-lignan flaxseed oil in the refrigerated section of your local health food store. I recommend mixing flaxseed oil in your salad dressing or into smoothies, green drinks, or even cottage cheese.

Dr. Johanna Budwig, a German biochemist, first brought attention to flaxseed oil as a cancer treatment back as the 1950s when she suggested mixing flaxseed oil with quark or cottage cheese. She argued that the unsaturated, high omega-3 fats in flaxseed oil, combined with the sulfur proteins of quark or cottage cheese, gave the body's cells the vital energy needed to fight cancer.[20]

The American Cancer Society says that most of the evidence for an anti-cancer effect of flaxseed and flaxseed oil stems from research using laboratory animals or cells grown in laboratory dishes. "In one culture study, flaxseed lignans reduced stickiness and movement of breast cancer cells . . . and researchers have also found that a diet supplement with flaxseed may reduce the formation, growth, or spread of prostate, breast, and skin cancer in mice," said the Web site.[21]

## Calcium

**Jordan:** Osteoporosis is a feared condition common for postmenopausal women, though men can suffer from bone loss as well. What happens is that with age, renewal of bone structure slows, causing bones to lose density and become more porous and brittle, creating a condition called osteoporosis.

The term *osteoporosis* literally means "porous bone," but doctors call it the "silent thief" because osteoporosis is an insidious condition that drains away bone mass so slowly, over many years, that many women are unaware that their bones have weakened considerably until there is a pronounced stoop in their posture or a fall resulting in a hip fracture. Osteoporosis leads to 1.5 million fractures per year, mostly in the hip, spine, and wrist, according to the National Institutes of Health. The condition afflicts 25 million Americans—80 percent of them older women. One of three women past the age of fifty will suffer a vertebral fracture because their bones are brittle.[22] Shrinking height is also a revealing sign of osteoporosis.

A number of factors come into play for the development of osteoporosis: a sedentary lifestyle, long-term use of certain medications, and a lack of minerals and hormones. There is no known cure for osteoporosis, which points to the importance of taking preventative measures to maintain—or at least slow—bone loss. Nutrition, as well as faithful exercise, is essential. Foods high in calcium, magnesium, and silica are needed for strong bones. Good dietary sources are green, leafy vegetables—available in green food supplements—cultured dairy products, sesame seeds, almonds, canned sardines, and salmon.

Remaining physically active aids bone density. Walking, a weight-bearing form of gentle exercise, deposits more minerals into the bones, especially the important skeletal frame that makes up the legs, hips, and spine. Unfortunately, a lack of exercise accelerates the loss of bone mass.

When it comes to supplements and osteoporosis, most people know that calcium gets the call. Every study I've seen over the years underscores the importance of calcium and bone health, including a *New England Journal of Medicine* study showing that taking calcium and vitamin D supplements tends to improve bone density and maintain strong bones and teeth.[23]

I've long viewed calcium as an "essential" ingredient because it's not naturally produced by the body and must be acquired through diet or supplements. (Another reason to eat foods that God created in a form that's healthy for the body.) The bones serve as the storage site for the body's calcium: if you don't get enough calcium through the foods you eat or the supplements you take, your body will drain it from your bones.

I recommend taking a whole food or "living" calcium containing magnesium, vitamin C, and vitamin D from whole food sources because they act together to give the bones physical structure, much like scaffolding put around a building renovation. Here's another situation where it's important to search for a *whole food* version of calcium instead of the regular commercial supplement.

These days, much of what passes for "calcium" is produced from ground-up rocks and even the shells of crustaceans—lobster, crabs, clams, and oysters. You can imagine how I feel about taking a supplement derived from an "unclean" source such as crustaceans. Our stomachs weren't designed to digest rocks or other inorganic substances, which are not readily absorbed by the body.

I believe the best calcium supplements are made with a combination of sea vegetables rich in calcium and microcrystalline hydroxyapatite, which is derived from the bones of free-range beef and lamb, two of the best sources of calcium. You should also look for whole food calcium supplements that contain vitamin C, vitamin D, iodine, zinc, magnesium, boron, copper, and manganese, which help the body properly absorb and utilize calcium. (To learn more about my favorite whole food calcium/magnesium complex, visit www.BiblicalHealthInstitute.com and click on the GPRx Resource Guide.)

### Antioxidants

Being married for seven years to Nicki has helped me realize that women take the health and appearance of their skin very seriously. So how do supplements fit in the mix?

They fit very well, thank you, because beauty starts on the inside. While women have long relied on creams and facials to maintain a peaches-and-cream complexion, supplements can play a role too. "In many ways, you can accomplish a lot more with supplements than you can with creams," said Zoe Diana Craelos, MD, an associate professor of dermatology at Wake Forest University.[24]

Dr. Craelos was referring to the powerful impact that antioxidants can have on your skin. Antioxidants are compounds that preserve and protect other compounds in the body from free-radical (oxygen-containing chemicals) damage. These unstable molecules are formed from sun exposure and pollutants in the air, and they destroy collagen, or the fibers that form the underlying support structure for your skin. "When this breakdown occurs, the skin shows signs of premature aging, including wrinkles, droops, and sags," wrote Colette Bouchez on the WebMD Web site. "Topical application of antioxidants is thought to block free-radical damage, and in this way preserve the integrity of our skin. But now experts say taking high levels *internally* can do even more."[25]

"Internally" means a healthy diet, with lots of vegetables, fruits, and whole grains, plus essential fatty acids from foods like omega-3 cod-liver and flaxseed oils. Unfortunately, as I've said before, we're not eating the way we should, and our foods don't pack the same nutritional punch as they did in a bygone era.

Taking antioxidants, like fruit and vegetable extracts, as well as extracts from coffee and teas, for beauty and skin care is another "cover your bases" idea, and one I support.

*What Women Are Saying*
*by Holly Wagner*

"The lump we removed from your breast was cancerous."

I was sure my doctor was not talking about me . . . this had to be a mistake. I mean, come on; I live in California, the land of sun and healthy people. I ate salads most every day and exercised every now and then, so this diagnosis just had to be wrong. Well, there was no mistake. I had joined a family of millions of women who were dealing with breast cancer.

Just days after hearing the diagnosis, a friend told me about this "amazing guy" named Rubin Jordan—or was it Jordan Rubin? She said Jordan's health plan was based on the Bible. I immediately bought his book and read it. Everything made sense. Even though I thought I had been living healthy, there were a number of changes I needed to make.

I have always been a little alternative in my approach to medicine. Sure, I would listen to advice from traditional oncologists, but I also wanted to look at everything I could do to strengthen my body and immune system. As I read Jordan's book, I realized that it was really no wonder my immune system was not functioning optimally. I had not been taking care of it.

So I made some changes. I immediately started taking whole food nutritional supplements. Perhaps in a perfect world, where the soil is full of nutrients, we wouldn't need supplements. But we don't live there, so we need them. I started taking enzymes and probiotics with SBOs. I significantly increased my green food intake and added a green superfood drink to my diet. I also increased the amount of water I drank. My digestive system has never worked better!

I also switched to organic produce and meat—no one's digestive system needs pesticides. And I ditched the pork and shellfish! If pork and shellfish are supposed to be the collectors of the earth's garbage, why would I want to eat them? It all began to make sense to me. God designed my body to be strong and healthy, and He had given me a plan to make that happen.

A month later, I underwent surgery as well as seven weeks of radiation. I stayed on the Great Physician's Rx the whole time and encountered very few side effects from the radiation. In fact, upon the conclusion of my treatments, my doctor looked at me and asked, "Did we radiate you?"

"Yes, you did." I grinned. Now I feel the best I've ever felt in my life, and for someone nearing the big 50, that ain't too shabby.

Not only will I follow this plan, but I will tell everyone I know that when they need a health tune-up, they should get a prescription from the Great Physician.

Holly Wagner, along with her husband, Philip, pastor the Oasis Christian Center in Los Angeles. She is the author of *When It Pours, He Reigns* and *God Chicks: Living Life as a 21st Century Woman.*

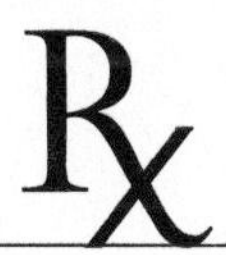

## THE GREAT PHYSICIAN'S Rx FOR WOMEN'S HEALTH: SUPPLEMENT YOUR DIET

- *Take a whole food living multivitamin with each meal.*
- *Consume a fiber/green food blend with flaxseed and beta glucans from soluble oat fiber each morning and evening.*
- *Consume one to three teaspoons or three to nine capsules of high omega-3 cod-liver oil per day with dinner.*
- *If you want improved digestion, take a probiotic and enzyme blend with each meal.*
- *Take a whole food calcium/magnesium blend with meals to maintain bone health, especially as you grow older and face osteoporosis.*

## THE GREAT PHYSICIAN'S RX FOR WOMEN'S HEALTH WEEK #2

Remember to visit www.BiblicalHealthInstitute.com and click on the GPRx Resource Guide to learn more about the foods and nutritional supplements recommended in the Great Physician's Rx 7 Weeks of Wellness plan.

### DAY 8

*You will notice that some items in the meal plans that follow are italicized. You can find the recipes for these—and over other 250 delicious and healthy recipes—at www.BiblicalHealthInstitute.com.*

***Upon Waking***

Drink 12 to 16 ounces of water.

***Breakfast***

During breakfast, drink 8 ounces of water.

two eggs (omega-3 or organic, prepared as desired)

one piece of fruit

one piece of whole-grain sprouted or sourdough toast with butter

hot tea with honey

*Supplements:* Take two whole food multivitamin caplets.

***Between Breakfast and Lunch***

Drink 12 ounces of water.

***Lunch***

During lunch, drink 8 ounces of water.

green salad with 3 ounces of grilled chicken and carrots, red onions, cucumbers, and yellow peppers

healthy salad dressing with 1 tablespoon of extra-virgin olive oil or high-lignan flaxseed oil

one piece of fruit

*Supplements:* Take two whole food multivitamin caplets.

***Between Lunch and Dinner***

Drink 12 ounces of water.

***Dinner***

During dinner, drink 8 ounces of water.

*Lemon Garlic Chicken*

pan-roasted, red bliss potatoes

steamed broccoli

*Supplements:* Take two whole food multivitamin caplets.

***Snack/Dessert***

apple cinnamon whole food bar (with beta-glucans from soluble oat fiber)

cottage cheese, fruit, and honey

## Day 9

*You will notice that some items in the meal plans that follow are italicized. You can find the recipes for these—and over other 250 delicious and healthy recipes—at www.BiblicalHealthInstitute.com.*

***Upon Waking***

*Supplements:* Take one serving of a fiber/green superfood combination containing ground flaxseed mixed in 12 to 16 ounces of water or raw vegetable juice.

***Breakfast***

During breakfast, drink 8 ounces of water.

For a healthy smoothie, mix the following in a blender:

8 ounces plain whole milk, yogurt, or kefir

1 tablespoon honey

1/2 cup fresh or frozen fruit (bananas, peaches, berries, pineapple, etc.)

1 teaspoon high-lignan flaxseed oil

1 serving of protein powder (optional)

*Supplements:* Take two whole food multivitamin caplets.

***Between Breakfast and Lunch***

Drink 12 ounces of water.

***Lunch***

During lunch, drink 8 ounces of water.

low-mercury, high omega-3 tuna on sprouted or yeast-free whole-grain bread with lettuce, tomato, and sprouts

one piece of fruit

*Supplements:* Take two whole food multivitamin caplets.

***Between Lunch and Dinner***

Drink 12 ounces of water.

***Dinner***

During dinner, drink 8 ounces of water.

fish of choice

sweet potato with butter

stir-fried veggies (onions, mushrooms, and peppers)

*Supplements:* Take two whole food multivitamin caplets.

***Snack/Dessert***

whole food meal replacement powder (with beta-glucans from soluble oat fiber) mixed in 12 ounces of water

cottage cheese, honey, and berries

***Before Bed***

*Supplements*: Take one serving of a fiber/green superfood combination containing ground flaxseed, mixed in 12 to 16 ounces of water or raw vegetable juice.

## DAY 10

*You will notice that some items in the meal plans that follow are italicized. You can find the recipes for these—and over other 250 delicious and healthy recipes—at www.BiblicalHealthInstitute.com.*

***Upon Waking***

*Supplements:* Take one serving of a fiber/green superfood combination containing ground flaxseed, mixed in 12 to 16 ounces of water or raw vegetable juice.

***Breakfast***

During breakfast, drink 8 ounces of water.

*Easy Oatmeal*

fried eggs

hot tea with honey

*Supplements:* Take two whole food multivitamin caplets.

***Between Breakfast and Lunch***

Drink 12 ounces of water.

***Lunch***

During lunch, drink 8 ounces of water.

green salad with 3 ounces of steak and carrots, red onions, cucumbers, and yellow peppers

healthy salad dressing with one tablespoon of extra-virgin olive oil or high-lignan flaxseed oil

one piece of fruit

*Supplements:* Take two whole food multivitamin caplets.

***Between Lunch and Dinner***

Drink 12 ounces of water.

***Dinner***

During dinner, drink 8 ounces of water.

*Chicken Fajitas*

green salad with red or yellow peppers, red onions, green or red cabbage, celery, cucumbers, and carrots

healthy salad dressing with olive oil and/or high-lignan flaxseed oil

*Supplements:* Take two whole food multivitamin caplets.

***Snack/Dessert***

berry antioxidant whole food bar (with beta-glucans from soluble oat fiber)

apple and almond or sesame butter (tahini)

***Before Bed***

*Supplements*: Take one serving of a fiber/green superfood combination containing ground flaxseed, mixed in 12 to 16 ounces of water or raw vegetable juice.

## DAY 11

*You will notice that some items in the meal plans that follow are italicized. You can find the recipes for these—and over other 250 delicious and healthy recipes—at www.BiblicalHealthInstitute.com.*

***Upon Waking***

*Supplements:* Take one serving of a fiber/green superfood combination containing ground flaxseed, mixed in 12 to 16 ounces of water or raw vegetable juice.

***Breakfast***

During breakfast, drink 8 ounces of water.

For a healthy smoothie, mix the following in a blender:

8 ounces plain whole milk, yogurt, or kefir

1 tablespoon honey

1/2 cup fresh or frozen fruit (bananas, peaches, berries, pineapple, etc.)

1 teaspoon high-lignan flaxseed oil

1 serving of protein powder (optional)

*Supplements:* Take two whole food multivitamin caplets and one capsule of omega-3 cod-liver oil.

***Between Breakfast and Lunch***

Drink 12 ounces of water.

***Lunch***

During lunch, drink 8 ounces of water.

turkey on sprouted or yeast-free whole-grain bread with lettuce, tomato, and sprouts

one piece of fruit

*Supplements:* Take two whole food multivitamin caplets and one capsule of omega-3 cod-liver oil.

***Between Lunch and Dinner***

Drink 12 ounces of water.

***Dinner***

During dinner, drink 8 ounces of water.

chicken dish of choice

green beans

*Supplements:* Take two whole food multivitamin caplets and one capsule of omega-3 cod-liver oil.

***Snack/Dessert***

whole food meal replacement powder (with beta-glucans from soluble oat fiber) mixed in 12 ounces of water

flax crackers, whole-grain crackers, or baked corn chips with salsa, hummus, or guacamole

***Before Bed***

*Supplements*: Take one serving of a fiber/green superfood combination containing ground flaxseed, mixed in 12 to 16 ounces of water or raw vegetable juice.

## DAY 12

*You will notice that some items in the meal plans that follow are italicized. You can find the recipes for these—and over other 250 delicious and healthy recipes—at www.BiblicalHealthInstitute.com.*

***Upon Waking***

*Supplements:* Take one serving of a fiber/green superfood combination containing ground flaxseed, mixed in 12 to 16 ounces of water or raw vegetable juice.

***Breakfast***

none (partial-fast day)

Drink 12 ounces of water.

***Between Breakfast and Lunch***

Drink 12 ounces of water.

***Lunch***

none (partial-fast day)

Drink 12 ounces of water.

***Between Lunch and Dinner***

Drink 12 ounces of water.

***Dinner***

During dinner, drink 8 ounces of water.

*Chicken Soup*

baked wild salmon

cultured vegetables

steamed green beans

green salad with red or yellow peppers, red onions, green or red cabbage, celery, cucumbers, and carrots

healthy salad dressing with olive oil and/or high-lignan flaxseed oil

*Supplements:* Take two whole food multivitamin caplets, one capsule of omega-3 cod-liver oil, and two caplets of a whole food calcium/magnesium blend.

### *Snack/Dessert*

none (partial-fast day)

### *Before Bed*

*Supplements:* Take one serving of a fiber/green superfood combination containing ground flaxseed, mixed in 12 to 16 ounces of water or raw vegetable juice.

## Day 13

*You will notice that some items in the meal plans that follow are italicized. You can find the recipes for these—and over other 250 delicious and healthy recipes—at www.BiblicalHealthInstitute.com.*

### *Upon Waking*

*Supplements:* Take one serving of a fiber/green superfood combination containing ground flaxseed, mixed in 12 to 16 ounces of water or raw vegetable juice.

### *Breakfast*

During breakfast, drink 8 ounces of water.

organic fresh ground coffee with organic cream and honey

one whole-grain pancake with maple syrup and butter

4 ounces of whole-milk yogurt with berries and honey, and 1/2 teaspoon of high-lignan flaxseed oil (optional)

*Supplements:* Take two whole food multivitamin caplets, one capsule of omega-3 cod-liver oil, and two caplets of a whole food calcium/magnesium blend.

***Between Breakfast and Lunch***

Drink 12 ounces of water.

***Lunch***

During lunch, drink 8 ounces of water.

green salad with raw cheese, avocado, walnuts, olives, carrots, red onions, cucumbers, and yellow peppers

healthy salad dressing with 1 tablespoon of extra-virgin olive oil or high-lignan flaxseed oil

one piece of fruit

*Supplements:* Take two whole food multivitamin caplets, one capsule of omega-3 cod-liver oil, and two caplets of a whole food calcium/magnesium blend.

***Between Lunch and Dinner***

Drink 12 ounces of water.

***Dinner***

During dinner, drink 8 ounces of water.

*Garlic Soup*

*Spaghetti and Meat Sauce*

spelt angel hair pasta

steamed broccoli

*Supplements:* Take two whole food multivitamin caplets, one capsule of omega-3 cod-liver oil, and two caplets of a whole food calcium/magnesium blend.

***Snack/Dessert***

green superfood whole food bar (with beta-glucans from soluble oat fiber)

soaked/sprouted, dehydrated nuts and seeds (crispy nuts)

***Before Bed***

*Supplements:* Take one serving of a fiber/green superfood combination containing ground flaxseed mixed in 12 to 16 ounces of water or raw vegetable juice.

## DAY 14

*You will notice that some items in the meal plans that follow are italicized. You can find the recipes for these—and over other 250 delicious and healthy recipes—at www.BiblicalHealthInstitute.com.*

***Upon Waking***

*Supplements:* Take one serving of a fiber/green superfood combination containing ground flaxseed, mixed in 12 to 16 ounces of water or raw vegetable juice.

***Breakfast***

During breakfast, drink 8 ounces of water.

two-egg omelet with avocado, cheese, tomato, onion, and pepper

*Sautéed Veggies*

hot tea and honey

*Supplements:* Take two whole food multivitamin caplets, one capsule of omega-3 cod-liver oil, and two caplets of a whole food calcium/magnesium blend.

***Between Breakfast and Lunch***

Drink 12 ounces of water.

***Lunch***

During lunch, drink 8 ounces of water.

almond butter and honey or pure fruit jam on sprouted or yeast-free whole-grain bread

one piece of fruit

*Supplements:* Take two whole food multivitamin caplets, one capsule of omega-3 cod-liver oil, and two caplets of a whole food calcium/magnesium blend.

***Between Lunch and Dinner***

Drink 12 ounces of water.

***Dinner***

During dinner, drink 8 ounces of water.

beef dish of choice

grilled onions, mushrooms, and peppers

green salad with red or yellow peppers, red onions, green or red cabbage, celery, cucumbers, and carrots

healthy salad dressing with olive oil and/or high-lignan flaxseed oil

*Supplements:* Take two whole food multivitamin caplets, one capsule of omega-3 cod-liver oil, and two caplets of a whole food calcium/magnesium blend.

***Snack/Dessert***

whole food meal replacement powder (with beta-glucans from soluble oat fiber) mixed in 12 ounces of water

*Banana Bread*

***Before Bed***

*Supplements*: Take one serving of a fiber/green superfood combination containing ground flaxseed mixed in 12 to 16 ounces of water or raw vegetable juice.

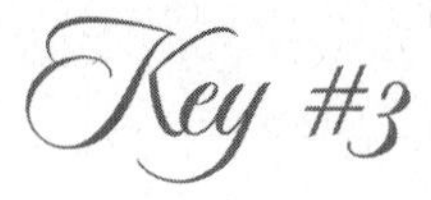

# Key #3

## *Practice Advanced Hygiene*

**Nicki:** I love Psalm 127:3: "Behold, children are a heritage from the LORD, the fruit of the womb is a reward" (NKJV). I've come to appreciate that verse as a young mother, but I shudder to think about millions of expectant women in centuries past, who approached looming childbirth with a measure of healthy respect and trepidation. In the eighteenth century, the chances of a birth ending in the mother's death—from infection, hemorrhage, convulsions, or dehydration—landed between 1 and 1.5 percent. This may not sound high, but since the typical mother gave birth to between five and eight children, her lifetime chance of dying in childbirth ran as high as one in eight. Put another way, if a mother in George Washington's time had eight female friends, she wasn't shocked if one of the expectant mothers died during childbirth. No wonder eighteenth-century women often referred to bringing a new life into the world as "the Dreaded apperation," "the greatest of earthly miserys," or "that evel hour I look forward to with dread."[1]

This morbid maternity situation didn't improve until a young doctor in Vienna, Austria, challenged medicine's conventional thinking on hygiene and the childbirth process. That doctor was Ignaz Semmelweis, who was born in Hungary in 1818, the fifth child of a prosperous German shopkeeper.

Just before he turned twenty, Ignaz traveled to Vienna to study law, but once in school, he was more attracted to medicine. He threw himself into his studies over the next seven years, completing his dissertation in 1844 and becoming a doctor. He applied for a position with the Vienna General Hospital, site of the world's largest maternity clinic, so he could learn from professor Johann Klein, a leading authority on puerperal fever, or what was known as "childbirth fever" in those days.

Though most women were still giving birth in their homes, more women were seeking medical attention for their "problem pregnancies." The problem, it turned out, was keeping mom and baby alive *after* the delivery. Mortality rates were ten, even twenty times higher inside the maternity ward than at home. Attending physicians scratched their heads and blamed the high death rate on crowded conditions or poor ventilation.

Within a year of arriving at Vienna General Hospital, Dr. Jakob Kolletschka, a close friend of Dr. Semmelweis, was performing an autopsy when he sliced his finger with a scalpel. An infection developed, and within days, Dr. Kolletschka died of symptoms resembling puerperal fever.

Dr. Semmelweis was beside himself. Why would his good friend die of puerperal fever? In a maternity clinic? That didn't make sense in a hospital with an international reputation for delivering babies, so Dr. Semmelweis began an investigation. The First Clinic, where physicians attended to upper-class mothers, had a dubious record: 13 percent of women or babies did not survive childbirth. Next door, at the Second Clinic, a second-class facility, where midwives delivered the babies, the mortality rate was 2 percent.

What Dr. Semmelweis noticed was that doctors left the dissection room and walked right into the delivery room, their hands practically dripping with the blood of cadavers. On a hunch and nothing more—Dr. Joseph Lister of Scotland wouldn't discover how to kill germs with heat and antiseptics for another eighteen years—Dr. Semmelweis established a new policy: from now on, doctors had to wash their hands in chlorinated water after working on cadavers. Within a month, the mortality rate from puerperal fever dropped from 13 to 2 percent.

What an amazing discovery! Or was it a coincidence? When word of Dr. Semmelweis's breakthrough made the rounds, he found himself caught in a political vise. His German boss, Dr. Klein, felt that he was being shown up by a young upstart—a Hungarian, no less!—so he blackballed him by blocking his promotion. The medical mainstream viewed Dr. Semmelweis as an outsider.

Downcast, the young doctor moved to Budapest, Hungary, where he accepted a position at a far more primitive hospital. Once again, he instituted a policy that doctors had to wash their hands in a chlorinated solution before delivering babies. The maternity clinic saw its mortality rate plunge to 1 percent.

This time, Dr. Semmelweis wrote a book about his discovery. Upon its release in 1861, the medical establishment circled their wagons and shot the messenger. Dr. Semmelweis fired back by writing several critical letters, which burned his bridges in the powerful Viennese medical community. Bitter about the lack of recognition and dogged in his determination that he was right, Dr. Semmelweis suffered a nervous breakdown. His family committed him to a private asylum in Vienna.

He died within two weeks under mysterious circumstances at the age of forty-seven. It's generally believed that Dr. Semmelweis passed away after becoming violent with asylum personnel, who beat him savagely. But the story persists—and here comes the interesting part—that he cut his finger and died of the same puerperal infection that had killed his friend Kolletschka and thousands of young mothers and their children during childbirth. Now, that's irony on the scale of a Greek tragedy.

Dr. Semmelweis was ahead of his time, but his pioneering work led to advances in hygiene, from which we all benefit today. These days, we take it as a matter of routine that our dentists and family physicians wash their hands before treating us. They have trained themselves to wash their hands and forearms thoroughly to rid the skin of infection-causing microorganisms.

I think about Dr. Semmelweis whenever I enter a public restroom and encounter someone who steps out of a stall and exits the facilities without washing her hands. What an appalling, disgusting, and all-too-common way to pass along germs to an unsuspecting public—you and me. While nothing is more fundamental to the human experience than using the bathroom, when you're done doing your business, you wash your hands. Elementary, my dear Watson.

In case you're saying to yourself that not washing one's hands is just a "guy thing," let me disabuse you of that notion. A major survey sponsored by the American Society of Microbiology (ASM) put observers in the restrooms of several major U.S. airports. I'm sure they didn't stand there with clipboards while people entered and exited, but they did note who washed their hands after using the facilities and who blew past them without bothering to pass their hands under a running faucet.

The tally after observing 7,541 travelers: 26 percent of males zipped up and bypassed the washbasin; but 17 percent of women also neglected to wash their hands after going to bathroom, results that astonish me because I'm a bit of a clean freak.[2] When I use a public restroom, I'll flush with my foot and scrub my hands with soap and water before drying them with a paper towel, which I also use to open the door. No way I'm reaching for a doorknob or handle that's been touched by who-knows-who with who-knows-what on her hands. Sometimes I have to put my foot in the door and stretch back as far as I can to drop the used paper towel in the trash, but if that's what it takes not to touch a dirty doorknob, I'll do it. (Many times I'll wipe the entire handle with the paper towel to help the next person out.)

There's no doubt that guys have it better, biologically speaking, when relieving themselves. For women, a trip to a public toilet—especially in an airplane—can become a test of gymnastic skills. I think every woman has hovered over a toilet at one time or another rather than let her bottom touch a seat teeming with critters. Even if you use disposable toilet seat covers, Waxies feel funny to the tush and have all the charm of a truck stop.

Floating over the toilet presents its own set of problems because the crouching position can prevent the bladder or bowel from emptying completely. Since women are at a physiological disadvantage compared to the men, no wonder public restrooms are nerve-wracking experiences.

### *A Fuselage Full of Germs at 35,000 Feet*
### *by Jordan Rubin*

I fly in and out of airports probably forty-eight weeks a year. It's absolutely brutal watching guys do their thing at the airport urinals and fail to wash up afterward, but after reading a San Diego State University study about airline bathrooms, I'm thinking about staying in my seat until I land.

San Diego State biology professor Scott Kelley took a small but scientific sampling of airline cleanliness in 2004, when participants swabbed surfaces at ten different places aboard various flights. They took biological evidence not only from armrests and tray tables, but toilet seats and handles, sinks, floors, unused paper towels, and doorknobs coming in and out of the planes' bathrooms.

After studying the microbial scuzz under a microscope, he determined that airline bathrooms were flying germ farms. "It was worse than a fraternity house in there," professor Kelley declared, referring to the toilets forward and aft. "I can't think of a more diverse area [of bacterial contamination]."[3] He discovered opportunistic pathogens like *Streptococcus, Staphylococcus, Cornybacterium, Proprionibacterium*, and *Kocuria* in his study published in the *Journal of Applied Microbiology*.[4]

Kelley said the situation doesn't warrant wearing surgical gloves the next time you board a flight, but he mentioned that whenever he flies and uses the facilities, he washes his hands well and uses a paper towel to open the lavatory door as he leaves.

The bathroom knob was the nastiest part of the plane, the researcher said.

**Jordan:** I feel sorry for women, especially when Port-o-Potties are the only ports of call. As for public restrooms, I've opened more doors with paper towels—or kicked them open—than I care to count.

More people are afraid of getting sick from germs in a public restroom than in any other place, according to a national survey conducted by Opinion Research Corporation. More than a thousand respondents said they were most likely to pick up germs in:

- public bathrooms (39 percent)
- restaurants (21 percent)
- airplanes (20 percent)

- subways and trains (11 percent)
- movie theaters (4 percent)[5]

**Nicki:** I can't believe hotel rooms weren't listed! When I'm in a hotel, you couldn't pay me to walk around barefoot. I have to wear slippers or shoes because I don't want my feet touching that dirty rug.

**Jordan:** I'm less concerned about walking barefoot on carpet because it's our hands—not our feet—that we need to be most concerned about. Our hands pick up germs from everything we touch: doorknobs, countertops, money, telephones, shopping carts, pens, and pencils. And those same hands pass along those germs to the next person. We're most vulnerable when we shake hands with others.

### *How Well Do You Know Germs?*

Chuck Gerba knows his germs.

Perhaps that's why this University of Arizona environmental-microbiology professor, who has devoted twenty-five years to researching this topic, is called "Dr. Germ" by his colleagues and the media.

So, based on the findings of one of his latest studies, which has the most germs: an ATM or a public restroom doorknob? A typical ATM touchpad, says Dr. Gerba, has more. Why? Because hands touching a public restroom doorknob are more likely to have been recently washed than those touching an ATM keypad.

What about a toilet seat in a fast food restaurant versus one on an airplane? Answer: the one on an airplane. Dr. Gerba says this can be attributed in part to the frequency with which restaurant toilets are cleaned, as compared to those on airplanes.

A Port-o-Potty, or a picnic table?

And the answer is . . . a picnic table. Sure, Port-o-Potties are gross, but Dr. Gerba says they are cleaned more frequently than picnic tables.

How did you do? Now I'm going to ask you three more questions:

1. Which place in the house has the most germs?
   - A. toilet bowl
   - B. garbage can
   - C. dishrag
   - D. refrigerator
   - E. bathroom doorknob
   - F. kitchen sink

The correct answer is C, the common dishrag. According to Dr. Gerba, the household kitchen is more heavily contaminated with bacteria than the bathroom. The dishrag and the kitchen sink are homes to the most germs, mainly because they stay moist most of the time.

2. Which place at work has the most germs?
   - A. elevator button
   - B. desktop
   - C. keyboard
   - D. phone receiver
   - E. toilet seat

Most people would say the toilet seat in the employee restroom, but the correct answer is D, the phone receiver. Toilet seats are cleaned more often with disinfectant than phone receivers, desktops, and keyboards.

3. Which public area has the most germs?
   - A. playground equipment
   - B. escalator handrails
   - C. shopping cart handles
   - D. Port-o-Potty
   - E. picnic table

It's not the picnic table this time. The correct answer is A, playground equipment.

When asked to explain the misconceptions, Dr. Gerba said, "Most people don't know where germs are."[6]

Germs *love* hands because once they establish a beachhead on your fingertips and under your nails, it's only a matter of time before you touch your lips, rub your eyes, scratch your nose, or itch your ears. Dr. Gerba says that the average adult touches his or her face one to three times every five minutes.[7] When—not if—the hand touches part of your face, bacteria are successfully transferred from your fingertips to one of these portals to your body. In the time it takes to sneeze, your body's immune system comes under attack.

**Nicki:** What's worse, women have another area of vulnerability: our reproductive anatomy. That's why we grow up learning that working out and getting our gym shorts and underwear sweaty—and not taking a shower and changing into new underwear and clothes right away—isn't a good idea. Bacteria and yeast love sweat, so when we don't change out of perspiration-soaked clothes, we're putting ourselves at risk for a urinary tract or yeast infection.

But personal hygiene is more than taking a shower after a workout. During our periods, we need to shower often, change tampons/sanitary napkins frequently, and always wash our hands before and after handling a tampon or pad. Some soaps can also irritate the delicate tissue of the vagina, which makes yeast infections more likely. Hygienists say we should use mild soap and unperfumed toilet paper, and cotton underwear is more sensible than tight thongs made from synthetic materials. (I'll talk more about personal hygiene products in Key #5.)

### *A Primer on Intimate Hygiene*
### *by Pancheta Wilson, MD*

Much of the advice I'm going to share you probably heard in your high-school sex ed class, but I've found that it's never a bad idea to offer a refresher course.

The female reproductive anatomy is one of God's most awesome creations, though some women grew up only hearing that their vaginas are dirty and germ filled. That's not true at all. Your vagina is naturally acidic and home to good bacteria that fight to keep bad bacteria out of your reproductive system. Most of the bacteria in the vagina are *Lactobacilli*, good bacteria that help keep out harmful bacteria and yeast from overgrowth. Certain conditions, however, predispose women to vaginal infections.

God has provided a mechanism by which the vagina naturally cleanses itself daily with a nonodorous clear or milky discharge. This fluid keeps the vagina healthy. A vaginal odor may result from a shift in the delicate balance between the organisms within the vagina, which results in an uncomfortable condition known as *bacterial vaginosis.*

Bacterial vaginosis and other vaginal infections require a trip to the gynecologist. Drinking plenty of water (another reason to drink six, seven, eight, or more glasses a day); using natural, healthy soap when you shower; and avoiding douches or commercial vaginal washes will help alleviate symptoms. Since the vagina is naturally clean and alive with healthy bacteria, washes, wipes, and sprays may interfere with the bacterial balance inside your vaginal canal. Douching kills off the protective bacteria, leaving your vagina vulnerable to attack from bad bacteria and increasing your risk for yeast infection.

Good hygiene begins with knowing the proper way to clean up after urination and defecation. Always wipe gently from the front to the back to prevent the spread of intestinal bacteria from the rectum to the urinary tract and vagina. Panty liners should be changed daily.

During puberty, you may have come home from school and discovered a watery or sticky stain of yellowish fluid on your underwear. You probably wondered what the fluid was—and may still wonder today. That fluid was estrogen, the hormone responsible for breast development and the start of menstruation. It also aids the body's natural defenses against infection. Vaginal secretions usually consist of water, albumin (an important protein in the body), and mucin—the smooth substance that gives the vagina and cervix a slippery texture.

Either way, do not scrub or use heavily perfumed soaps or sprays on your vaginal area. Instead, cleanse with clean water when you shower or bathe. When you shave around the genital area, realize that shaving can cause ingrown hairs, rashes, and nicks to the skin, which increase the risk of infection.

And if you use bikini wax treatments, be aware that some professional salons don't clean up the way they should; therefore, you could be exposing yourself to bacteria left behind from recent clients.

**Jordan:** No way I'm getting within an area code of this discussion. At any rate, the most important thing about hygiene is washing your hands. It is *the* single most important act of personal hygiene. It's also your strongest line of defense against cold and flu viruses, as well as other potentially dangerous germs. Teaching—and reminding—your children to wash their hands frequently not only keeps them from getting sick, but it could prevent them from passing along the latest flu bug to *you.*

**Nicki:** Or maybe something worse than a flu bug. I've changed a couple of thousand diapers in the last two years, including an average of two poopy diapers a day, so I have no problem scrubbing my hands after each time I clean my little guy. I mean, *Hello!* No way would I handle or prepare food for the next meal without a thorough hand washing. It would be unthinkable for me to do so.

I'm just as conscientious when I'm out of the house. I've mentioned how I use a paper towel to open restroom doors, but I keep packets of baby wipes in my purse to use when Joshua and I visit a grocery store or one of those big toy stores because there are a lot of germs lurking on the handles of those shopping carts. I don't want Joshua touching cart handles because he's like any toddler who puts his fingers in his mouth and wipes the gooey hands everywhere, but that's impossible for a toddler.

Shopping carts, though incredibly helpful, happen to be incredibly dirty. The Korea Consumer Protection Board found that shopping-cart handles are the most bacteria-infested item in a list of commonly touched objects, averaging 1,100 colony-forming units (CFU) of bacteria per square meter. (Internet café computer mouses, bus hand straps, and public toilet doorknobs are two, three, and four.)[8]

I'm happy to report that Publix supermarkets here in my home state of Florida provide free disinfectant wipes at store entrances so shoppers can wipe down their handles before heading down the grocery aisles or putting Junior in his little seat. Still, whenever I've been grocery shopping, I wash my hands. It is important to always do so when you've been in public. Here are some other occasions when you should remind yourself to wash your hands:

- before and after you insert and remove contact lenses
- before eating, especially if you're eating something with your hands, like a sandwich
- after you sneeze, cough, or blow your nose
- after cleaning up a dog's mess
- after blowing your child's nose
- after handling garbage
- after cleaning up the kitchen sink and nearby countertops
- after cleaning a bathroom
- after shaking a lot of hands at church
- after doing errands, especially shopping at a supermarket
- after attending an event at a public theater
- after making love

It's not necessary to place your hands under scalding hot water to wash your hands; warm water will suffice. Apply a generous dollop of semisoft soap and rub your hands together vigorously, working the soap into and under your fingernails, especially if they are long. You should rub and scrub for fifteen to thirty seconds, or about the time it takes to slowly sing "Happy Birthday to Me." If you're in a public restroom that doesn't have automatic faucets, use a paper towel in your hand to turn off the running water. Also use a paper towel to open the door. Finally, keep waterless sanitizers in your purse to use the next time soap and water aren't available in a public restroom, or to wipe off a shopping-cart handle.

**Jordan:** It is vital that hand washing be practiced by *everyone.* Why? The fingertips are repositories of germs because tiny microbes lodge in the soft tissue under your fingernails. Every time you touch your face, your immune system is susceptible to attack. Germs, once inside your body, explode in numbers and go after healthy cells like rampaging Vikings. Before you can say, "I think I'm coming down with something," your nose runs like the Mississippi, your throat is scratchy as sandpaper, and you're sneezing like a circus clown trying to get a big laugh.

Maybe you haven't paid attention to how easily germs enter the body through the nasal passageway or the corners of the eyes—the tear ducts—when you touch those areas. All of us rub our faces so often that we don't even know we're doing it half the time, but when skin-on-skin or skin-on-membrane contact is made, you transfer a garden variety of bacteria, allergens, environmental toxins, and viruses from one part of the body to another. In medical terms, it's called auto- or self-inoculation of the conjunctival (the eyes) or nasal (the nose) mucosa with a contaminated finger.

According to Australian scientist Kenneth Seaton, PhD, ear, nose, and throat problems—which represent 80 percent of visits to doctors' offices—can be linked to the fact that humans inoculate their noses, eyes, mouths, and skin with dirty fingernails throughout the day. He estimates that 90 percent of the germs hide underneath your fingernails, no matter how short you keep them trimmed.

Dr. Seaton, who has studied hygiene since the late 1950s, said that the conventional wisdom in medical circles is that colds and influenza are mainly spread by germs and viruses swirling through the air after one has coughed or sneezed in close proximity. Thus, prevention was thought to be almost impossible because who can protect themselves from airborne exposure? "For years, I struggled to educate and convince the medical establishment that hand transmission is by far the most efficient mechanism for spreading germs and viruses," said Dr. Seaton.[9]

The Australian scientist was convinced that germs were much more likely to be spread by hand-to-hand contact than by airborne exposure. To test his theory, he conducted a research study in which ten healthy people shared a large room with ten other people suffering from an active virus. They were told they had to stay there for eight hours. They could talk, eat, and read, but the healthy subjects were not allowed to touch those who were sick. When the eight hours were up, Dr. Seaton and his researchers tested the ten healthy people. Two of the ten had caught the virus.

The next time, Dr. Seaton repeated his study with ten healthy people walking into a large room with ten sick people. Again, they were told they could do what they wanted, but this time, no restrictions were put on physical contact with one another. After eight hours, every single healthy person was getting sick because he or she had been infected with the virus through touching. Thus, people were five times more likely to be infected by picking up a virus via hand-to-hand transmission than by someone's sneeze sending germs through the air. The results prompted Dr. Seaton to coin the axiom "Germs don't fly; they hitchhike."

I've been influenced a great deal by the research of Dr. Seaton, who said that advanced hygiene techniques are the single most important factor in maintaining good health. "All the vitamins, minerals, herbs, special diets, and exercise machines pale in comparison to hygiene. The Spartans in ancient Greece exercised to perfection, practiced the best possible diet, had no pollution and little stress, yet life expectancy was around twenty-six years of age," he wrote in his newsletter, *Hygiene & Health*. "Their society perished because of its failure to adopt good personal hygiene techniques."

What do those techniques look like? Since 90 percent of germs take up residence around my fingernails, I use a creamy semisoft soap rich in essential oils. Each morning and evening, I dip both hands into the tub of semisoft soap and dig my fingernails into the cream. Then I work the special cream around the tips of my fingers, cuticles, and fingernails for fifteen to thirty seconds. When I'm finished, I lather my hands for fifteen seconds before rinsing them under running water. After my hands are clean, I take another scoop of semisoft soap and wash my face. My second step involves a procedure that I call a "facial dip." I fill my washbasin or a clean, large bowl with warm but not hot water. Then I add one to two tablespoons of regular table salt and two eyedroppers of a mineral-based facial solution into the cloudy water. I mix everything up with my hands, and then I bend over and dip my face into the cleansing matter, opening my eyes several times to allow the membranes to be cleansed. After coming up for air, I dunk my head a second time and blow bubbles through my nose. "Sink snorkeling," I call it.

My final two steps of advanced hygiene involve applying very diluted drops of hydrogen peroxide and minerals into my ears for thirty to sixty seconds to cleanse the ear canal, followed by brushing my teeth with an essential oil–based tooth solution to cleanse my teeth, gums, and mouth of unhealthy germs.

Following this advanced hygiene protocol involves discipline; you have to remind yourself to do it until it becomes an ingrained habit. I find it easier to follow these steps in the morning when I'm freshly awake rather than later in the evening, when I'm tired and bleary eyed, though I do my best to practice advanced hygiene morning and evening. Either way, I know it takes only three minutes or so to complete all of the steps.

The most important step in advanced hygiene is washing your hands often. While we don't run the risk of dying from nineteenth-century diseases like puerperal fever, we still risk getting sick. I've been following this advanced hygiene protocol ever since I learned about it ten years ago, when I was very sick. Since then, I've been virtually illness-free from the usual respiratory ailments and sinus infections that afflict millions of Americans each day. All it takes is three minutes twice a day—once in the morning and once at bedtime—to practice advanced hygiene in the privacy of your own bathroom.

*Clean Thoughts About the Act of Love*
*by Pancheta Wilson, MD*

Another aspect of hygiene that should be addressed deals with the privacy of your bedroom. Obviously, lovemaking is the most intimate behavior between a married couple, but sexual contact also involves extensive use of the fingers at times. Additionally, bodily fluids are exchanged, which is why personal hygiene before and after sexual activity cannot be overemphasized. You can practice advanced hygiene by taking a shower before sexual intimacy, paying special attention to your fingers and nails. This is especially important for your husband since he will be touching you in your most intimate areas.

Notice I said "your husband." That's because God created sex to be enjoyed *between a husband and a wife.* The Bible is clear: "Honor marriage, and guard the sacredness of sexual intimacy *between wife and husband.* God draws a firm line against casual and illicit sex" (Heb. 13:4 MSG, emphasis added). When we stray *outside* God's guidelines, sexual contact can become a life-and-death issue.

Within the confines of a monogamous marriage, the transfer of a sexually transmitted disease (STD) is nil—if the couple waited until marriage to begin sexual activity. But if you are not married and are engaged in sexual activity, your actions can lead to disaster. Unfortunately, premarital sex is the norm in today's "hook-up" generation. People casually enter and exit sexual relationships as though they were passing through a revolving door. The result is a huge increase in sexually transmitted diseases. Genital herpes is labeled a silent killer, and it's estimated that 45 million Americans are infected, with up to one million new cases each year, according to the U.S. Department of Health and Human Services.[10] Many people have such mild cases that they are unaware of the presence of infection, which means they infect others without having a clue.

Then there are a host of other STDs: bacterial vaginosis, chlamydia, genital warts, gonorrhea, HIV, human papillomavirus, syphilis, and trichomoniasis. Many STDs lead to conditions such as pelvic inflammatory disease, cervical cancer, and complications in pregnancy. And everyone knows about the scourge of AIDS.

Couples who engage in unclean sexual practices will unfortunately reap what they sow. Take the practice of heterosexual anal sex. Tim and Beverly LaHaye, authors of *The Act of Marriage After 40*, took this issue head-on, and I agree with what they say:

> There is one sexual act that we do not favor: anal intercourse. We don't believe God made our bodies for that practice, and the anus doesn't serve a sexual purpose for the body. That act, known as sodomy, is highly dangerous for both partners. Once inside the anus, the penis can become contaminated with disease-producing organisms, thus causing dangers to the man's reproductive and urinary structures.[11]

Not to mention the danger to the woman if the man proceeds from anal to vaginal intercourse.

God did not make any mistakes when He created our bodies; there is no way to be clean when participating in unclean sexual practices.

**Nicki:** I practice advanced hygiene, but I'm not as faithful as Jordan, and I wish I were. I usually follow the advanced hygiene regimen once a day—and more often when I feel a cold coming on. I have no trouble motivating myself to follow this program when we fly together because I know that advanced hygiene helps me ward off colds and sicknesses that I used to get on plane rides. (Learning about dirty airplane bathrooms in this chapter doesn't inspire confidence, either.)

The reason I don't practice advanced hygiene as often as Jordan is because I'm usually home most of the day, where I'm caring for Joshua and able to wash my hands regularly. Jordan, on the other hand, travels a great deal and is constantly meeting people and shaking hands. It's not uncommon for him to shake a few hundred hands after he speaks at a church on Sunday morning or does a book signing at a Barnes and Noble. I know the first thing he does when he gets back to the hotel is to thoroughly wash his hands by dipping them into a semisoft soap so he can remove germs from underneath his fingernails.

Which prompts a random question to pop up in my head: Should pastors invite the congregation to shake hands with each other? Not to get paranoid about the topic, but sometimes in January and February, when it seems like half the church is hacking away during the pastor's sermon, I've asked myself that question because I know that there are active flu viruses sticking their thumbs out so they can hitchhike a ride into my immune system. During the Spanish flu epidemic of 1918–1919, when an estimated 670,000 Americans perished, some cities passed ordinances making it illegal to shake hands.[12]

To answer my own question, I think pastors should continue the practice of inviting everyone to say hello or introduce themselves, although I can understand why priests in the Roman Catholic diocese of Metuchen, New Jersey, advised parishioners that they had the option to smile, bow, or wave instead of shaking hands with neighbors.[13] Unless I have a cold, I'll shake a hand that's offered to me. I meet a lot of people, especially when I'm with Jordan, so I think it would be *worse* not to shake someone's hand. So I shake the hand, and then I wash my hands afterward.

**Jordan:** We've been talking a lot about the importance of washing your hands often, but there's another orifice to be concerned about—the ears. Back in 1928, Dr. Richard Simmons—not the fitness guru; he's not that old—hypothesized that cold and flu germs can sneak into the body through the ear canal. Dr. Joseph Mercola of mercola.com advises administering a few drops of 3 percent hydrogen peroxide ($H_2O_2$) into each infected ear when cold and flu symptoms present themselves. There may be some bubbling or mild stinging in the ear canal, but hydrogen peroxide, a household antiseptic used on cuts and scrapes, loosens packed earwax, and its powerful oxidizing qualities kill bacteria and viruses. (Note: never attempt to clean your ears aggressively before having them examined by your doctor.)

Finally, there's a protein floating around in your body that you should know about, and it happens to be the most abundant one. It's called albumin, and it transports hormones and nutrients in your bloodstream and moves waste out. Like dump trucks on their way to the landfill, albumin hauls wastes and toxic cells to the liver for degradation and elimination from the body.

Your risk of catching a cold or flu shoots way up when albumin levels in the blood go down. Dr. Seaton is certain that poor hygiene causes albumin levels to drop because the immune system can't produce enough to defend the body when under attack by cold and flu viruses. Albumin levels can be optimized by practicing advanced hygiene, which underscores the importance of this key as part of the Great Physician's Rx for women's health.

*What Women Are Saying*
*by Holly Covington*

My health issues, related to a hormonal imbalance made evident by very infrequent periods, began when I was thirteen. As I got into my twenties, I gained weight unexplainably and couldn't lose it no matter what I did or tried. By my late twenties, I was having debilitating, crippling headaches almost every day.

For almost ten years, I went to doctors, trying to get answers, but this is what they told me:

"There's nothing the matter with you."

"You're just feeling stress."

"We can't find anything wrong with you."

But I knew in my heart that something was wrong with me. It couldn't be normal to wake up in the morning, feeling pain before I even opened my eyes.

It was hard to be a mother to my children and a wife to my husband when I felt so poorly and was experiencing so much pain. Finally, I was diagnosed with polycystic ovarian syndrome (PCOS), as well as prediabetes, and went on multiple medications, which only helped to a point.

My husband, Tom, and I had been praying to God to show us a way to get my health back. One night we had dinner with my sister, Sherri, who had been given a copy of Jordan's book at church that previous Sunday. She gave it to me to read in hopes that it would help. All it took was one hour reading Jordan's book to know that I had to try the Great Physician's Rx.

Shopping for healthy food was a culture shock. I went to stores that I had never visited before and purchased foods I had never eaten—good foods, organic foods. I got into the advanced hygiene program, which cleared up my sinus problems. Later my daughter got a severe case of conjunctivitis, which caused her eyes to swell shut and ooze horrible green stuff. When I showed her how to practice advanced hygiene, her eye problems were gone by the morning.

As for Key #4 and getting physically fit, I didn't have time to go to the gym because I take care of my two children and my two nieces during the day, so I have four kids vying for my attention. But when I learned about functional fitness, that was something I could do when the kids were playing or taking a nap. Let me tell you, doing functional fitness for just five minutes a day made a big difference in my physical appearance.

How big a difference? In the first twelve days of eating foods that God created and doing functional fitness exercises, I lost eight and a half pounds. After ten months, I had lost thirty pounds; eight inches in my waist, stomach, and thighs; and two to three dress sizes.

My health has improved so much that I'm a different person. I'm off all medications for the first time since Tom and I got married. I have more energy and vitality, my thinking is sharper and clearer, and I no longer wake up with pain, which is a great way to start the day.

## Rx THE GREAT PHYSICIAN'S Rx FOR WOMEN'S HEALTH: PRACTICE ADVANCED HYGIENE

- *Dip your fingers into a semisoft soap with essential oils and wash your hands several times a day, paying special attention to removing germs from beneath your fingernails. Teach your children to do the same.*
- *Cleanse your nasal passageways and the mucous membranes of the eyes daily by performing a facial dip.*
- *Cleanse the ear canals several times per week.*
- *Use an essential oil-based tooth solution daily to remove germs from the teeth, gums, and mouth.*
- *Remind your children that viruses and bacteria are all over desks, doorknobs, and computer keyboards at school. Describe how easy it is for them to transport those germs from their hands to their mouths, eyes, and noses.*
- *Do not douche or use heavily perfumed soaps or sprays on your vaginal area.*
- *Practice sexual hygiene, and avoid anal intercourse.*

## The Great Physician's Rx for Women's Health Week #3

Remember to visit www.BiblicalHealthInstitute.com and click on the GPRx Resource Guide to learn more about the foods and nutritional supplements recommended in the Great Physician's Rx 7 Weeks of Wellness plan. You can also find more than 250 healthy and delicious recipes, including the italicized recipes in this chapter, at this site.

### Day 15

*You will notice that some items in the meal plans that follow are italicized. You can find the recipes for these—and over other 250 delicious and healthy recipes—at www.BiblicalHealthInstitute.com.*

**Upon Waking**

*Advanced hygiene:* For hands and nails, Jab fingers into semisoft soap four or five times, and lather them for fifteen seconds, rubbing soap over cuticles and rinsing under water as warm as you can stand. Take another scoop of semisoft soap into your hands, and wash your face.

*Supplements:* Take one serving of a fiber/green superfood combination containing ground flaxseed, mixed in 12 to 16 ounces of water or raw vegetable juice.

**Breakfast**

During breakfast, drink 8 ounces of water.

two eggs (omega-3 or organic, prepared as desired)

one piece of fruit

one piece of whole-grain sprouted or sourdough toast with butter

hot tea with honey

*Supplements:* Take two whole food multivitamin caplets, one capsule of omega-3 cod-liver oil, and two caplets of a whole food calcium/magnesium blend.

**Between Breakfast and Lunch**

Drink 12 ounces of water.

***Lunch***

During lunch, drink 8 ounces of water.

green salad with two hard-boiled omega-3 eggs, carrots, red onions, cucumbers, and yellow peppers

healthy salad dressing with one tablespoon of extra-virgin olive oil or high-lignan flaxseed oil

one piece of fruit

*Supplements:* Take two whole food multivitamin caplets, one capsule of omega-3 cod-liver oil, and two caplets of a whole food calcium/magnesium blend.

***Between Lunch and Dinner***

Drink 12 ounces of water.

***Dinner***

During dinner, drink 8 ounces of water.

*Spinach and Goat Cheese Meat Lasagna*

green salad with red or yellow peppers, red onions, green or red cabbage, celery, cucumbers, and carrots

healthy salad dressing with olive oil and/or high-lignan flaxseed oil

*Supplements:* Take two whole food multivitamin caplets, one capsule of omega-3 cod-liver oil, and two caplets of a whole food calcium/magnesium blend.

***Snack/Dessert***

apple cinnamon whole food bar (with beta-glucans from soluble oat fiber)

whole-milk yogurt, fruit, and honey

***Before Bed***

*Supplements:* One serving of a fiber/green superfood combination containing ground flaxseed, mixed in 12 to 16 ounces of water or raw vegetable juice

*Advanced hygiene:* for hands and nails, jab fingers into semisoft soap four or five times, and lather hands with soap for fifteen seconds, rubbing soap over cuticles and rinsing under water as warm as you can stand. Take another swab of semisoft soap into your hands and wash your face.

## DAY 16

*You will notice that some items in the meal plans that follow are italicized. You can find the recipes for these—and over other 250 delicious and healthy recipes—at www.BiblicalHealthInstitute.com.*

### *Upon Waking*

*Advanced hygiene:* for hands and nails, jab fingers into semisoft soap four or five times, and lather hands with soap for fifteen seconds, rubbing soap over cuticles and rinsing under water as warm as you can stand. Take another swab of semisoft soap into your hands and wash your face. Next, fill basin or sink with water as warm as you can stand, and add one to three tablespoons of table salt and one to three eyedroppers of iodine-based mineral solution. Swirl water. Dunk face into water and open eyes, blinking repeatedly.

*Supplements:* Take one serving of a fiber/green superfood combination containing ground flaxseed, mixed in 12 to 16 ounces of water or raw vegetable juice.

### *Breakfast*

During breakfast, drink 8 ounces of water.

For a healthy smoothie, mix the following in a blender:

8 ounces plain whole milk, yogurt, or kefir

1 tablespoon honey

1/2 cup fresh or frozen fruit (bananas, peaches, berries, pineapple, etc.)

1 teaspoon high-lignan flaxseed oil

1 serving of protein powder (optional)

*Supplements:* Take two whole food multivitamin caplets, one capsule of omega-3 cod-liver oil, and two caplets of a whole food calcium/magnesium blend.

### *Between Breakfast and Lunch*

Drink 12 ounces of water.

### *Lunch*

During lunch, drink 8 ounces of water.

Low-mercury, high omega-3 tuna on sprouted or yeast-free whole-grain bread with lettuce, tomato, and sprouts

one piece of fruit

*Supplements:* Take two whole food multivitamin caplets, one capsule of omega-3 cod-liver oil, and two caplets of a whole food calcium/magnesium blend.

***Between Lunch and Dinner***

Drink 12 ounces of water.

***Dinner***

During dinner, drink 8 ounces of water.

*EZ Pizza*

green salad with red or yellow peppers, red onions, green or red cabbage, celery, cucumbers, and carrots

healthy salad dressing with olive oil and/or high-lignan flaxseed oil

*Supplements:* Take two whole food multivitamin caplets, one capsule of omega-3 cod-liver oil, and two caplets of a whole food calcium/magnesium blend.

***Snack/Dessert***

whole food meal replacement powder (with beta-glucans from soluble oat fiber) mixed in 12 ounces of water

one piece of fruit and 1 ounce of cheese

***Before Bed***

*Supplements:* One serving of a fiber/green superfood combination containing ground flaxseed, mixed in 12 to 16 ounces of water or raw vegetable juice

*Advanced hygiene:* for hands and nails, jab fingers into semisoft soap four or five times, and lather hands with soap for fifteen seconds, rubbing soap over cuticles and rinsing under water as warm as you can stand. Take another swab of semisoft soap into your hands and wash your face.

Next, fill basin or sink with water as warm as you can stand, and add one-to-three tablespoons of table salt and one-to-three eyedroppers of iodine-based mineral solution. Swirl water. Dunk face into water and open eyes, blinking repeatedly underwater.

## Day 17

*You will notice that some items in the meal plans that follow are italicized. You can find the recipes for these—and over other 250 delicious and healthy recipes—at www.BiblicalHealthInstitute.com.*

### *Upon Waking*

*Advanced hygiene:* for hands and nails, jab fingers into semisoft soap four or five times, and lather hands with soap for fifteen seconds, rubbing soap over cuticles and rinsing under water as warm as you can stand. Take another swab of semisoft soap into your hands and wash your face.

Next, fill basin or sink with water as warm as you can stand, and add one-to-three tablespoons of table salt and one-to-three eyedroppers of iodine-based mineral solution. Swirl water. Dunk face into water and open eyes, blinking repeatedly underwater.

*Supplements:* Take one serving of a fiber/green superfood combination containing ground flaxseed, mixed in 12 to 16 ounces of water or raw vegetable juice.

### *Breakfast*

During breakfast, drink 8 ounces of water.

sprouted dried cereal with yogurt, kefir, goat's milk, or almond milk

banana

hot tea with honey

*Supplements:* Take two whole food multivitamin caplets, one capsule of omega-3 cod-liver oil, and two caplets of a whole food calcium/magnesium blend.

### *Between Breakfast and Lunch*

Drink 12 ounces of water.

### *Lunch*

During lunch, drink 8 ounces of water.

green salad with 3 ounces of tuna (low-mercury, high omega-3) and carrots, red onions, cucumbers, and yellow peppers healthy salad dressing with 1 tablespoon of extra-virgin olive oil or high-lignan flaxseed oil

one piece of fruit

*Supplements:* Take two whole food multivitamin caplets, one capsule of omega-3 cod-liver oil, and two caplets of a whole food calcium/magnesium blend.

***Between Lunch and Dinner***

Drink 12 ounces of water.

***Dinner***

During dinner, drink 8 ounces of water.

fish of choice

baked sweet potato

green salad with red or yellow peppers, red onions, green or red cabbage, celery, cucumbers, and carrots

healthy salad dressing with olive oil and/or high-lignan flaxseed oil

*Supplements*: Take two whole food multivitamin caplets, one capsule of omega-3 cod-liver oil, and two caplets of a whole food calcium/magnesium blend.

***Snack/Dessert***

berry antioxidant whole food bar (with beta-glucans from soluble oat fiber)

apple with almond or sesame butter (tahini)

***Before Bed***

*Supplements:* Take one serving of a fiber/green superfood combination containing ground flaxseed, mixed in 12 to 16 ounces of water or raw vegetable juice.

*Advanced hygiene:* for hands and nails, jab fingers into semisoft soap four or five times, and lather hands with soap for fifteen seconds, rubbing soap over cuticles and rinsing under water as warm as you can stand. Take another swab of semisoft soap into your hands and wash your face.

Next, fill basin or sink with water as warm as you can stand, and add one-to-three tablespoons of table salt and one-to-three eyedroppers of iodine-based mineral solution. Swirl water. Dunk face into water and open eyes, blinking repeatedly underwater.

## DAY 18

*You will notice that some items in the meal plans that follow are italicized. You can find the recipes for these—and over other 250 delicious and healthy recipes—at www.BiblicalHealthInstitute.com.*

*Upon Waking*

*Advanced hygiene:* for hands and nails, jab fingers into semisoft soap four or five times, and lather hands with soap for fifteen seconds, rubbing soap over cuticles and rinsing under water as warm as you can stand. Take another swab of semisoft soap into your hands and wash your face.

Next, fill basin or sink with water as warm as you can stand, and add one-to-three tablespoons of table salt and one-to-three eyedroppers of iodine-based mineral solution. Swirl water. Dunk face into water and open eyes, blinking repeatedly underwater. (This time, keep eyes open underwater for three seconds.) After cleaning your eyes, put your face back in the water, and close your mouth while blowing bubbles out of your nose.

*Supplements:* Take one serving of a fiber/green superfood combination containing ground flaxseed, mixed in 12 to 16 ounces of water or raw vegetable juice.

*Breakfast*

During breakfast, drink 8 ounces of water.

For a healthy smoothie, mix the following in a blender:

8 ounces plain whole milk, yogurt, or kefir

1 tablespoon honey

1/2 cup fresh or frozen fruit (bananas, peaches, berries, pineapple, etc.)

1 teaspoon high-lignan flaxseed oil

1 serving of protein powder (optional)

*Supplements:* Take two whole food multivitamin caplets, one capsule of omega-3 cod-liver oil, and two caplets of a whole food calcium/magnesium blend.

*Between Breakfast and Lunch*

Drink 12 ounces of water.

***Lunch***

During lunch, drink 8 ounces of water.

turkey on sprouted or yeast-free whole-grain bread with lettuce, tomato, and sprouts

one piece of fruit

*Supplements*: Take two whole food multivitamin caplets, one capsule of omega-3 cod-liver oil, and two caplets of a whole food calcium/magnesium blend.

***Between Lunch and Dinner***

Drink 12 ounces of water.

***Dinner***

During dinner, drink 8 ounces of water.

*Chicken with Sun-Dried Tomatoes and Spinach*

roasted red potatoes

peas and carrots

*Supplements:* Take two whole food multivitamin caplets, one capsule of omega-3 cod-liver oil, and two caplets of a whole food calcium/magnesium blend.

***Snack/Dessert***

whole food meal replacement powder (with beta-glucans from soluble oat fiber) mixed in 12 ounces of water

raw veggies and hummus, salsa, or guacamole

***Before Bed***

*Supplements:* Take one serving of a fiber/green superfood combination containing ground flaxseed, mixed in 12 to 16 ounces of water or raw vegetable juice.

*Advanced hygiene:* for hands and nails, jab fingers into semisoft soap four or five times, and lather hands with soap for fifteen seconds, rubbing soap over cuticles and rinsing under water as warm as you can stand. Take another swab of semisoft soap into your hands and wash your face.

Next, fill basin or sink with water as warm as you can stand, and add one-to-three tablespoons of table salt and one-to-three eyedroppers of iodine-based mineral solution. Swirl water. Dunk face into water and open eyes, blinking repeatedly underwater.

Swirl water. Dunk face into water and open eyes, blinking repeatedly underwater. Keep eyes open underwater for three seconds. After cleaning your eyes, put your face back in the water, and close your mouth while blowing bubbles out of your nose.

## DAY 19 (PARTIAL-FAST DAY)

*You will notice that some items in the meal plans that follow are italicized. You can find the recipes for these—and over other 250 delicious and healthy recipes—at www.BiblicalHealthInstitute.com.*

***Upon Waking***

*Advanced hygiene:* for hands and nails, jab fingers into semisoft soap four or five times, and lather hands with soap for fifteen seconds, rubbing soap over cuticles and rinsing under water as warm as you can stand. Take another swab of semisoft soap into your hands and wash your face.

Next, fill basin or sink with water as warm as you can stand, and add one-to-three tablespoons of table salt and one-to-three eyedroppers of iodine-based mineral solution. Swirl water. Dunk face into water and open eyes, blinking repeatedly underwater. Keep eyes open underwater for three seconds. After cleaning your eyes, put your face back in the water, and close your mouth while blowing bubbles out of your nose.

*Supplements:* Take one serving of a fiber/green superfood combination containing ground flaxseed, mixed in 12 to 16 ounces of water or raw vegetable juice.

***Breakfast***

none (partial-fast day)

Drink 12 ounces of water.

***Between Breakfast and Lunch***

Drink 12 ounces of water.

***Lunch***

none (partial-fast day)

Drink 12 ounces of water.

***Dinner***

During dinner, drink 8 ounces of water.

*Chicken Soup*

*Wood-Grilled King Salmon*

sautéed asparagus

cultured vegetables

green salad with red or yellow peppers, red onions, green or red cabbage, celery, cucumbers, and carrots

healthy salad dressing with olive oil and/or high-lignan flaxseed oil

*Supplements:* Take two whole food multivitamin caplets, one capsule of omega-3 cod-liver oil, and two caplets of a whole food calcium/magnesium blend.

***Snacks***

Drink 12 ounces of water.

***Before Bed***

*Supplements:* Take one serving of a fiber/green superfood combination containing ground flaxseed mixed in 12 to 16 ounces of water or raw vegetable juice.

*Advanced hygiene:* for hands and nails, jab fingers into semisoft soap four or five times, and lather hands with soap for fifteen seconds, rubbing soap over cuticles and rinsing under water as warm as you can stand. Take another swab of semisoft soap into your hands and wash your face.

Next, fill basin or sink with water as warm as you can stand, and add one-to-three tablespoons of table salt and one-to-three eyedroppers of iodine-based mineral solution. Swirl water. Dunk face into water and open eyes, blinking repeatedly underwater. Keep eyes open underwater for three seconds. After cleaning your eyes, put your face back in the water, and close your mouth while blowing bubbles out of your nose. Come up from the water, and immerse your face in the water once again, gently taking water into your nostrils and expelling bubbles. Come up from the water, and blow your nose into facial tissue.

## DAY 20

*You will notice that some items in the meal plans that follow are italicized. You can find the recipes for these—and over other 250 delicious and healthy recipes—at www.BiblicalHealthInstitute.com.*

### *Upon Waking*

*Advanced hygiene:* for hands and nails, jab fingers into semisoft soap four or five times, and lather hands with soap for fifteen seconds, rubbing soap over cuticles and rinsing under water as warm as you can stand. Take another swab of semisoft soap into your hands and wash your face.

Next, fill basin or sink with water as warm as you can stand, and add one-to-three tablespoons of table salt and one-to-three eyedroppers of iodine-based mineral solution. Swirl water. Dunk face into water and open eyes, blinking repeatedly underwater. Keep eyes open underwater for three seconds. After cleaning your eyes, put your face back in the water, and close your mouth while blowing bubbles out of your nose. Come up from the water, and immerse your face in the water once again, gently taking water into your nostrils and expelling bubbles. Come up from the water, and blow your nose into facial tissue.

Next, to cleanse the ears, use hydrogen peroxide and mineral-based ear drops, putting two or three drops into each ear and letting stand for sixty seconds. Tilt your head to expel the drops.

*Supplements:* Take one serving of a fiber/green superfood combination containing ground flaxseed, mixed in 12 to 16 ounces of water or raw vegetable juice.

### *Breakfast*

During breakfast, drink 8 ounces of water.

sprouted or raw, dry cereal

4 ounces of whole-milk yogurt or goat's milk

raw honey

fresh fruit

hot tea with honey

*Supplements:* Take two whole food multivitamin caplets, one capsule of omega-3 cod-liver oil, and two caplets of a whole food calcium/magnesium blend.

***Between Breakfast and Lunch***

Drink 12 ounces of water.

***Lunch***

During lunch, drink 8 ounces of water.

green salad with 3 ounces of salmon and carrots, red onions, cucumbers, and yellow peppers

healthy salad dressing with one tablespoon of extra-virgin olive oil or high-lignan flaxseed oil

one piece of fruit

*Supplements:* Take two whole food multivitamin caplets, one capsule of omega-3 cod-liver oil, and two caplets of a whole food calcium/magnesium blend.

***Between Lunch and Dinner***

Drink 12 ounces of water.

***Dinner***

During dinner, drink 8 ounces of water.

*Chicken Soup*

steamed broccoli

green salad with red or yellow peppers, red onions, green or red cabbage, celery, cucumbers, and carrots

healthy salad dressing with olive oil and/or high-lignan flaxseed oil

*Supplements:* Take two whole food multivitamin caplets, one capsule of omega-3 cod-liver oil, and two caplets of a whole food calcium/magnesium blend.

*Snack/Dessert*

green superfood whole food bar (with beta-glucans from soluble oat fiber)

*Zesty Popcorn* with butter and spices

*Before Bed*

*Supplements:* Take one serving of a fiber/green superfood combination containing ground flaxseed, mixed in 12 to 16 ounces of water or raw vegetable juice.

*Advanced hygiene:* for hands and nails, jab fingers into semisoft soap four or five times, and lather hands with soap for fifteen seconds, rubbing soap over cuticles and rinsing under water as warm as you can stand. Take another swab of semisoft soap into your hands and wash your face.

Next, fill basin or sink with water as warm as you can stand, and add one-to-three tablespoons of table salt and one-to-three eyedroppers of iodine-based mineral solution. Swirl water. Dunk face into water and open eyes, blinking repeatedly underwater. Keep eyes open underwater for three seconds. After cleaning your eyes, put your face back in the water, and close your mouth while blowing bubbles out of your nose. Come up from the water, and immerse your face in the water once again, gently taking water into your nostrils and expelling bubbles. Come up from the water, and blow your nose into facial tissue. To cleanse the ears, use hydrogen peroxide and mineral-based ear drops, putting two or three drops into each ear and letting stand for sixty seconds. Tilt your head to expel the drops.

## DAY 21

*You will notice that some items in the meal plans that follow are italicized. You can find the recipes for these—and over other 250 delicious and healthy recipes—at www.BiblicalHealthInstitute.com.*

*Upon Waking*

*Advanced hygiene:* for hands and nails, jab fingers into semisoft soap four or five times, and lather hands with soap for fifteen seconds, rubbing soap over cuticles and rinsing under water as warm as you can stand. Next, fill basin or sink with water as warm as you can stand, and add one-to-three tablespoons of table salt and one-to-three eyedroppers of iodine-based mineral solution. Swirl water. Dunk face into water and open eyes, blinking repeatedly underwater. Keep eyes open underwater for three seconds. After cleaning your eyes, put your face back in the water, and close your mouth while blowing bubbles out of your nose.

Come up from the water, and immerse your face in the water once again, gently taking water into your nostrils and expelling bubbles. Come up from the water, and blow your nose into facial tissue. To cleanse the ears, use hydrogen peroxide and mineral-based ear drops, putting two or three drops into each ear and letting stand for sixty seconds. Tilt your head to expel the drops.

For the teeth, apply two or three drops of essential oil–based tooth drops to the toothbrush. This can be used to brush your teeth or can be added to existing toothpaste. After brushing your teeth, brush your tongue for fifteen seconds.

*Supplements:* Take one serving of a fiber/green superfood combination containing ground flaxseed, mixed in 12 to 16 ounces of water or raw vegetable juice.

***Breakfast***

During breakfast, drink 8 ounces of water.

two-egg omelet with avocado, cheese, tomato, onion, and pepper

*Sautéed Veggies*

hot tea and honey

*Supplements:* Take two whole food multivitamin caplets, one capsule of omega-3 cod-liver oil, and two caplets of a whole food calcium/magnesium blend.

***Between Breakfast and Lunch***

Drink 12 ounces of water.

***Lunch***

During lunch, drink 8 ounces of water.

almond butter and honey or pure fruit jam on sprouted or yeast-free whole-grain bread

one piece of fruit

*Supplements:* Take two whole food multivitamin caplets, one capsule of omega-3 cod-liver oil, and two caplets of a whole food calcium/magnesium blend.

***Between Lunch and Dinner***

Drink 12 ounces of water.

***Dinner***

During dinner, drink 8 ounces of water.

chicken dish of choice

green salad with red or yellow peppers, red onions, green or red cabbage, celery, cucumbers, and carrots

healthy salad dressing with olive oil and/or high-lignan flaxseed oil

*Supplements:* Take two whole food multivitamin caplets, one capsule of omega-3 cod-liver oil, and two caplets of a whole food calcium/magnesium blend.

***Snack/Dessert***

whole food meal replacement powder (with beta-glucans from soluble oat fiber) mixed in 12 ounces of water

*Blueberry Muffins*

***Before Bed***

*Supplements:* Take one serving of a fiber/green superfood combination containing ground flaxseed, mixed in 12 to 16 ounces of water or raw vegetable juice.

*Advanced hygiene:* for hands and nails, jab fingers into semisoft soap four or five times, and lather hands with soap for fifteen seconds, rubbing soap over cuticles and rinsing under water as warm as you can stand. Take another swab of semisoft soap into your hands and wash your face.

Next, fill basin or sink with water as warm as you can stand, and add one-to-three tablespoons of table salt and one-to-three eyedroppers of iodine-based mineral solution. Swirl water. Dunk face into water and open eyes, blinking repeatedly underwater. Keep eyes open underwater for three seconds. After cleaning your eyes, put your face back in the water, and close your mouth while blowing bubbles out of your nose.

Come up from the water, and immerse your face in the water once again, gently taking water into your nostrils and expelling bubbles. Come up from the water, and blow your nose into facial tissue. To cleanse the ears, use hydrogen peroxide and mineral-based ear drops, putting two or three drops into each ear and letting stand for sixty seconds. Tilt your head to expel the drops. For the teeth, apply two or three drops of essential oil–based tooth drops to the toothbrush. This can be used to brush your teeth or added to existing toothpaste. After brushing your teeth, brush your tongue for fifteen seconds.

# *Key #4*

## *Condition Your Body with Exercise and Body Therapies*

**Nicki:** When we visited the Yorkeys in Switzerland, Jordan and I landed at Zurich's Kloten Airport, where Mike and Nicole were waiting for us. Nearly all air travel from the U.S. to Europe involves overnight flights, so when we landed at 8 a.m. local time, my body groaned since it was still on Eastern Standard Time—two o'clock in the morning. I hadn't slept a wink.

Nicole proposed taking the scenic route from Zurich to the family chalet in Villars. Instead of driving the more direct path on the fast *autobahn*, she said we could detour on secondary roads that would lead us through the heart of the Swiss Alps—the Interlaken region, home to Heidi and the majestic Eiger Mountain.

I wish I could say that I was stunned by the beauty of the Brünig Pass, which gave us our first glimpse of the Eiger's North Face, still snowcapped on this September morning. I wish I could tell you about the magnificent chalets constructed from Norwegian pinewood and accented with window boxes that overflowed with white, orange, and blood-red geraniums. I wish I could describe the coral-blue Thunersee, a glacier-fed lake teeming with windsurfers and pleasure boaters on that Sunday morning.

But I was fast asleep in our rental car. Jordan conked out for most of the trip as well. No matter how hard I tried, I couldn't keep my eyes open during the five-hour journey.

After arriving in Villars, our hosts recommended that we take a short walk to "keep you two going." Getting some fresh air gave us a burst of energy and kept us engaged during dinner, a delicious dinner of Swiss fondue—wedges of organic *pain rustique* dipped into a bubbling mixture of Gruyère and Vacherin cheeses. But we tired quickly and turned in early. At 8:30 p.m., after tucking myself beneath a dreamy duvet, I fell into a deep sleep the moment my jet-lagged head hit the fluffy pillow.

I was dead to the world.

Jordan woke up thirteen glorious hours later and enjoyed a late-morning breakfast with the Yorkeys. At 11 a.m., he wondered if he should interrupt my slumber. Nicole, a mother who knows that you never wake up a sleeping child—or mom—demurred. "Let her sleep," she said.

At 2:00, Mike suggested we start a March Madness–like pool on when I would wake up. Thirty minutes later, it was apparent that I wasn't going to wake up anytime in the near future. If I didn't get up *now*, they reasoned, then I might sleep past dinnertime, and then I would be really messed up.

Finally, Jordan walked into our bedroom, making noise and opening the shutters. Bright sunlight filled the room, and I came to life.

"You've been sleeping for eighteen hours," Jordan said though a drowsy haze.

*Eighteen hours.* That was a new world record—at least for me. After I brought baby Joshua home from the hospital, there were *weeks* during which I didn't sleep more than eighteen hours. Grabbing that much sleep in a Swiss chalet felt like a guilty pleasure, but I deserved it after what I had been through for the last year and a half. Like most breastfeeding mothers, during Joshua's first six months of life, I never snoozed longer than spurts of three or four hours. Many times I was so exhausted that I couldn't fall back asleep after a middle-of-the-night feeding.

After dozing eighteen hours in the Swiss Alps, I felt as though I was making up, in a small way, for eighteen sleep-deprived *months* back home in Florida. Every mother feels a sense of exhaustion, which stems from not getting enough sleep and the tyranny of the urgent: taking care of the kids and tackling too many things around the house. If you're a young mother like me, then finding a full night of rest is an elusive pipe dream, even though we know that sleep is a basic human need, as important to good health as what we eat and how much we exercise.

Whether you have kids or not, and whatever age you are, sleep lays the groundwork for a productive day ahead, it's important for women to wake up to the importance of sleep. I know I can tell the difference when I get to bed early and squeeze out an extra hour of wonderful sleep. Adequate rest revitalizes tired bodies, gives us more energy, helps us think more clearly throughout the day, and puts us in better moods. So why don't women get more bed rest?

Because we're too busy! I've come to a point where getting enough sleep just isn't in the cards, though there are steps we can and should take to sleep better and a little longer. I understand that for mothers of toddlers or infants, sleep will always be a rationed commodity. I'm waiting until Joshua gets older, when I hope to sleep longer than six hours and forty-one minutes per night, the national average for women between the ages of thirty and sixty, according to the National Sleep Foundation's Women and Sleep poll.[1]

**Jordan:** Six hours and forty-one minutes isn't enough rest, but sleep is a body therapy in short supply these days. This chapter will discuss body therapies—which range from sleep to exercise, from saunas to sunning yourself—the fourth key that will unlock your health potential.

Nicki and I harbor no illusions that we're getting enough sleep at night; we're among the millions of droopy-eyed parents packing in as much as we can from the instant our feet hit the floor to the moment we crawl under the covers sixteen, seventeen, or eighteen exhausting hours later. I would say that we average between six and seven hours a night. I can assure you, that is not enough sleep for good health.

I wish we could snatch eight hours, which is the magic number, sleep experts say. (When people are allowed to sleep as much as they would like in a controlled setting, such as a sleep laboratory, they naturally sleep eight hours in a twenty-four-hour time period.)

**Nicki:** I guess I'll have to catch up on my rest in heaven. What Jordan and I have been doing in the last year is taking small steps, like going to bed earlier on occasion. Some evenings we've turned in shortly after 10 p.m., which I believe is an ideal time in today's fast-paced world. We used to go to bed and watch meaningless news programs for an hour and a half before turning off the TV and the lights at 11:30, but no longer. Now we make it a priority to go to bed without watching TV, which has made a big difference in how rested we feel when Joshua lets us know that he's ready to tackle the day—sometime around 5:30 to 6 a.m.

Another thing I've done to improve my sleep, especially when Jordan is out of town on business, is exercise before I retire. I'm not talking about going to the gym or running around the block. What I do is a few "functional exercises" that Jordan taught me (which he will describe soon in greater detail). Raising my heart rate and extending myself physically tires me out—and makes me sleep better. When Jordan is home, we also like to read the Bible and pray together before saying good night.

### *The Dangers of Sleep Medications*
### *by Pancheta Wilson, MD*

In my practice, lots of women complain about not getting enough sleep, which they usually want me to fix that day—I mean, that *night.* They say they can't turn their minds off, or they can't fall asleep, so they lie awake most of the night. Others lie awake beside their husbands, with eyes closed but listening to his every inhale and exhale of breath, wondering why they cannot fall asleep and stay asleep.

Insomnia, which affects more than 70 million Americans, according to the National Institutes of Health, is medically defined by these four descriptors:

- difficulty falling asleep, especially within thirty minutes of lying down
- waking up frequently during the night, and difficulty returning to sleep
- waking up too early in the morning and sleeping less than six and a half hours over a typical night
- unrefreshing sleep[2]

Insomnia is experienced by both males and females in all age groups, but it seems to be more common in women, especially after menopause.[3] Physicians used to view insomnia as a symptom that something was off-kilter in the patient's life, but new evidence suggests that insomnia may not be a symptom of other conditions but rather a disorder in its own right.

Physicians generally approach the treatment of chronic insomnia with one of three options. The first includes behavioral therapy, which may involve working with a psychologist or psychiatrist. Another form of behavioral therapy applies to stimulus control, which trains couples to use their beds and bedrooms for sleep and sex only.

Nearly all of my insomnia patients request the third option—a prescription for a sleep medication. Patients these days are savvy enough to ask for them by name—Ambien, Sonata, or Lunesta—which only validates the power of mass-media advertising. This trio of sleep medications is part of a third generation of sleeping pills that evolved from anesthetic agents in the 1950s. They are extremely sedating and can cause problems if too high a dose is given. Hollywood's Marilyn Monroe slipped into a coma caused by an alleged overdose of sleeping pills.

The next breakthrough in sleeping pills originated from a drug called *flurazepam* and marketed as Dalmane. These sleeping pills are derivatives of Valium.[4] Over the past decade, we've seen a third wave of sleeping pills that are effective without the sedating or addicting qualities of the older versions. Ambien comes with a quickly dissolving outer layer meant to immediately induce sleep and a slower-dissolving inner layer to sustain sleep. About 42 million sleep prescriptions were filled in 2005, according to the research company IMS Health, up nearly 60 percent since 2000.[5]

I resist handing out prescriptions for sleep medication in a carte blanche manner. Instead, I recommend a more natural approach to getting a good night's rest. I suggest herbal teas, infusions, and baths, which have calming effects. As a Christian physician, I'm able to offer prayer for healing and deliverance to those patients who want it. One of my patients, a fellow physician, informed me that prayer works better than any pill! My own personal experience is that since I became born-again and spirit-filled, I sleep like a baby.

*Prescription for Nutritional Healing* recommends eating bananas, dates, figs, tuna, whole-grain crackers, yogurt, or turkey—foods high in sleep-promoting tryptophan—before going to bed.[6] (And you always wondered why you got sleepy after a big Thanksgiving dinner.) The nutritional supplement, melatonin, is a hormone that promotes sleep and is popular among those averse to taking a prescription sleep medication.

If your husband snores, I suggest he be tested for sleep apnea. Meanwhile, if his snoring bothers you, then you may want to try a device that covers up the noise. Some women are said to have good success with a sound machine that creates a wall of white noise or the chirping of crickets to block out the noise pollution from heavy sleepers. It may be worth it to check out the Homedics Sound Spa, which is billed as an "acoustic relaxation machine," producing six soothing sounds that range from summer crickets to waves breaking on a beach.

When I don't feel like exercising at bedtime, I often listen to Christian books on tape by authors Perry Stone or John Hagee. The thing I *won't* do is take a pill or medication to cause me to sleep. I've noticed the alluring ads for Ambien and Lunesta, but I've never taken one of those meds, and I don't see myself ever starting. I wasn't big on the indiscriminate use of medications such as sleeping pills before I met Jordan, so it doesn't make sense to me to start now. I was also wary of the possible side effects, long- and short-term.

**Jordan:** As you would expect, I would never ingest a prescription pill to help me fall asleep, either, but Nicki mentioned something that's very important to unlocking this fourth key to your health potential: exercise. Physical fitness is essential to good health and is one of the best things you can do for your body, mind, and spirit. Exercise does a body good; pumping those legs and arms speeds up the heart and makes you breathe faster, which helps transfer oxygen from your lungs to your blood and increases the body's natural virus-killing cells. Exercise stimulates the disease-fighting white blood cells in the body to move from the organs into the bloodstream, where they can mount a defense against those germs that enter the body's portals, which we examined in the last chapter.

Exercise contributes to mental health as well. New research suggests that physical exercise encourages healthy brains to function at their optimal levels. When lab animals exercise, their nerve cells release chemicals called *neurotrophic factors*, explained an article in *Science News* magazine. "Out of the variety of neurotrophic factors released during exercise, however, scientists found that one in particular stood out: brain-derived neurotrophic factor, or BDNF," said the article. "This protein seems to act as a ringleader, both prompting brain benefits on its own and triggering a cascade of other neural health-promoting chemicals to spring into action."[7] Translation: You feel better about yourself. You experience a rise in self-esteem and a reduction in stress. I saw this happen time and time again as a certified fitness trainer. Even a simple walk on a treadmill may provide an immediate mood lift.

In another study done at the University of Texas at Austin, researchers compared the effects of thirty minutes of walking on a treadmill with thirty minutes of quiet rest in forty adults recently diagnosed with depression. None of the participants were exercising regularly. While the results showed that both groups reported reductions in feelings of tension, anger, depression, and fatigue, only the exercise group reported a greater sense of well-being and vigor.[8]

The point of Key #4 is that regular exercise—starting with just five minutes and working up to fifteen, twenty, or thirty minutes a day at least five days a week—can help a woman live a healthy lifestyle, prevent her from getting sick, and lift her mood. My favorite way to get the body moving is called *functional fitness*, a form of gentle exercise that raises the heartbeat, strengthens the body's core muscles, and exercises the cardiovascular system through the performance of real-life activities in real-life positions.

Functional fitness can be done by using body weight only or by employing dumbbells, mini trampolines, and stability balls. When Nicki wants to exercise before bed, she'll pick up some ten-pound barbells and put herself through a set of motions and rotations. She uses a stability ball to strengthen her abs. Many of the functional fitness exercises can be performed without weights. If you want to use weights, though, and you don't have any free weights at home, you can always use sixteen-ounce cans of tomato sauce.

### *A Sample Functional Fitness Program by Jordan Rubin*

If I were leading a functional fitness class in your living room, I'd have you do my four favorite functional fitness movements to make you stronger and more flexible:

- **Alternate overhead press.** Begin by standing with your feet shoulder-width apart. Keeping your midsection straight, fully extend your right arm, with the palm facing up, as if pushing a box skyward. As your right arm comes down, make the same motion with the left arm, palm up. Start with five repetitions for each arm, building up to ten or twenty. You can "press" a small can of canned vegetables to get stronger.
- **Bicep curl.** Here's another easy one. Take both arms and stretch them out at your thighs with both hands facing down. Curl each arm, one at a time, bending only at the elbow, for a set of ten. A more advanced position would be pulling one elbow up to shoulder height and making a motion similar to pulling a lawnmower starting cord.
- **Squats.** This is an exercise that you don't want to do if the last time you performed a squat was in junior-high gym class. If you're game, though, stand with your feet shoulder-width apart. Squat down as far as you comfortably can, with your arms stretched out for balance and your palms facing down. A more advanced squat would include holding dumbbells or a medicine ball while you dip toward the ground. Do twenty of these, and you'll be feeling the burn.
- **Lunges.** There's a reason this exercise is popular in aerobic classes—it's harder than it looks! Technique is important, as it is for all these functional exercises. Keep the back leg straight when you lunge forward with one large step. You also want the knee directly over the ankle with each lunge; otherwise, you're stepping too far.

If you can get away from the house or office, you can find functional fitness classes and equipment at gyms around the country, including LA Fitness, Bally Total Fitness, and local YMCAs. You'll raise your heartbeat with an assortment of squats, lunges, push-ups against a wall, and "supermans," which involve lying on the floor and lifting up your right arm while lifting your left leg into a fully extended position. (For more information on functional fitness, visit www.BiblicalHealthInstitute.com.)

But I don't have time for any classes. And, to be perfectly honest, I don't like to exercise. I think many women feel the same.

I wasn't always this way. Growing up, I enjoyed exercising, ran cross-country at my high school for three years, and after college, I jogged three miles a day, five times a week, to stay in shape. And I loved working out with Jordan in the gym when we met. I'm afraid I've lost the desire to exercise, especially after my son was born. I really have to force myself do it, even though functional fitness is much more fun than other forms of exercise.

**Jordan:** That's what I love about my wife—she's honest, says what's on her heart. She's in a different season of life right now, a loving mother focused on the needs of a little one totally dependent on her. She takes stroller walks with Joshua, though she prefers to drive to a nearby air-conditioned mall instead of walking in muggy, strength-sapping Florida heat. We both enjoy our after-dinner walks around a nearby lake in our neighborhood.

This goes to show you that there are alternatives to joining a gym. Walking is a form of gentle exercise that requires no expensive outlay of cash. You can walk whenever it fits into your schedule: the crack of dawn before work, during a morning break, over the lunch hour, before dinner, after a meal, or in the twilight hours. You can go at your own pace, and it's an exercise that you can do every day. It's also a superb social activity since walking is tailor-made for talking at the same time. Moms pushing strollers together is a great way to combine physical activity with social interaction.

The whole idea behind walking is to perform steps, and the more steps, the better. Just ask the Amish. Researcher David R. Bassett Jr., professor of exercise science at the University of Tennessee, put pedometers on ninety-eight Amish adults and learned that the men averaged 18,000 steps a day and performed ten hours of vigorous physical activity a week (heavy lifting, shoveling or digging, tossing hay bales, etc.). Women averaged 14,000 steps a day and three and a half hours of vigorous physical activity a week.[9] This level of exertion goes a long way toward explaining why obesity in the Amish community ranks at a paltry 4 percent, as compared to a third of American adults.

"The average American accumulates 3,000 to 5,000 steps per day," said Bassett.[10] But the goal, say experts, should be 10,000 steps a day. Hearing about this has revolutionized the way I think: when I'm taking the stairs instead of the elevator, I'm adding steps to my day. (I think I'll ask Nicki for a pedometer for my birthday.)

**Nicki:** When Jordan isn't traveling, he often watches Joshua so that I can go to the gym. Although my first inclination is to say no because I have other things to do, a little voice reminds me that I always feel better after a workout.

*Excuses, Excuses*
*by Jordan Rubin*

It's amazing how nimble the mind is when it comes to creating rationalizations to keep us away from a date with exercise. I'm going to offer a collection of common excuses, followed by my counterpoint:

*Excuse:* "I'm too busy."
*Counterpoint:* Sure, you are. My life is insanely busy as well. But unless you schedule exercise—treat it like an appointment—it will always remain unchecked on your "to do" list.

*Excuse:* "I don't have the time."
*Counterpoint:* You will if you introduce functional fitness into your life.

Functional fitness can be performed in as little as five minutes, whereas many exercise programs involve exercising one hour a day, three times a week, or half an hour for five or six days a week. And I'm not even including the time it takes to drive to the local gym. Furthermore, for some odd reason, people who exercise regularly seem to get more done in a day, not less.

*Excuse:* "I don't have the energy."
*Counterpoint:* That's probably because you don't exercise. Try exercising before work. The endorphin rush will lift your day.

*Excuse:* "I can't get up that early."
*Counterpoint:* You can if you go to bed thirty minutes earlier.

*Excuse:* "I'm too fat."
*Counterpoint:* You'll weigh less if you start exercising.

*Excuse:* "It costs too much money to join a fitness club."
*Counterpoint:* It costs too much *not* to exercise. Remember: if you don't have your health, you don't have anything—and that will cost you *everything.*

*Excuse:* "It's too cold."
*Counterpoint:* If you're working out at home or at a fitness club, I'm sure it's heated.

*Excuse:* "It's too hot."
*Counterpoint:* Try living in Florida. We have air-conditioning in the Sunshine State, and I'm sure your fitness club does too.

*Excuse:* "It's been so long since I exercised."
*Counterpoint:* So? A thousand-mile journey begins with a single step.

*Excuse:* "There's something good on TV."
*Counterpoint:* Then tape the show for later viewing. TiVo anyone?

*Excuse:* "I can't get motivated."
*Counterpoint:* Then find a friend who'll exercise with you. It's harder to break an exercise appointment with a partner than when you're exercising alone.

*Excuse:* "If I exercise, I'll eat too much."
*Counterpoint:* People who exercise are more likely to eat *well*, and people who eat well are more likely to exercise.

Women are busy, and usually something has to give. The last thing they have time for is exercise. But once most people—and I'm including guys in this—cross off exercise from their "to do" lists, they're left with three choices:

1. play the martyr and pretend they're victims and can't exercise;
2. figure there's always tomorrow to get out there and break a sweat; or
3. try to do *something* physically active, which has lifelong implications.

The best choice is, of course, the third one. Playing the martyr is a self-fulfilling prophecy, and promising yourself that you'll exercise tomorrow is just procrastination. Choosing to do some type of exercise—and figuring out a way to get that done—means choosing to raise your quality of living and get your body in shape for the long haul. Because life really is for the long haul.

**Jordan:** Although exercising adds another time commitment to your busy day, it doesn't seem to create *more* stress. David Nieman, an Appalachian State University researcher, put a control group of "stressed-out" women (as determined by psychological testing) on a brisk walking program. After a month of walking, he tested them against a sedentary control group and found that the walking women "maintained an elevated mood."[11]

Exercise is a rewarding pastime that reduces your risk of dying prematurely (especially from heart disease, the number-one killer for women), decreases your chance of developing high blood pressure, lessens feelings of depression and anxiety, diminishes stress in your life, and helps control your weight. Exercises also builds and maintains healthy bones, muscles, and joints—the best preventive measure you have against osteoporosis. Finally, exercise promotes psychological well-being and improves your mood, which impact your relationships with your family and close friends.

So what will it take for you to exercise twenty to thirty minutes, five times a week? Purchasing a treadmill and walking on it while you catch up on the news after work? (Don't lug a home treadmill into the laundry room; it's guaranteed to become a glorified clothesline.) Starting a walking club with some of your senior friends? Is it screening an aerobics video and raising your heartbeat while your toddler takes his first nap of the day? Is it preparing dinner before your husband arrives home from work and then letting him watch the little ones while you go to the gym or embark on a long walk around the neighborhood?

*Breaking a Sweat?*
*by Jordan Rubin*

Instead of a purchasing a treadmill, which can be expensive and take up a lot of room, consider a rebounder instead. These minitrampolines work great with functional fitness because you can begin with five or ten minutes of functional fitness exercises and finish with five or ten minutes with a rebounder. Yes, it takes good balance to jump repeatedly on a rebounder, but you'll see results quickly. Many rebounders come with videos that you can follow while you exercise, or you can play your favorite music in the background; just make sure it has a good beat. Rebounders strengthen muscles, tendons, and ligaments and help bones become dense and strong. Women with knee problems like rebounders because they are landing their feet on a soft surface as opposed to an unforgiving surface like a sidewalk or asphalt street. And you don't have to buy an expensive rebounder from one of the TV infomercials. You can buy a minitrampoline for under $40 at most large merchandise stores.

Any of these options take discipline, and I've found that morning is the best time to exercise, if for no other reason than you can't cancel a workout that you've already finished. A morning workout is also great due to the sense of accomplishment it brings you throughout the day. If the morning doesn't work, then choose a time that works for you because your body is capable of exercising at any hour. But mornings are best, and then you can rest.

## REST AND RELAXATION

**Nicki:** Can someone define the words *rest* and *relaxation* for me? These days when I hear the words *rest* and *relaxation* in the same sentence, I'm thinking *spa.* Not that I've been to one lately, but checking into a full-service spa for some pampering sounds like a great idea. But since lingering in a mud bath with slices of cucumber over my eyes is a daydream, I'll have to be content with snatching some relaxing moments whenever I can. As of right now, my favorite way to chill is in our home sauna.

We live in Florida, where people do their darndest to *escape* the heat, not get into it, but Jordan was the one who got introduced to saunas and something called hydrotherapy, which initially sounded like another one of his radical ideas. Hydrotherapy, he explained, was when you made use of hot or cold water for therapeutic reasons. For instance, hydrotherapy could be as simple as an extended bath in a tub of hot water and soapy suds, submerging your body as well as your troubles under a blanket of soothing heat.

Another way to experience hydrotherapy is by immersing yourself in a backyard pool and experiencing a kind of weightlessness similar to an astronaut being relieved of the pull of gravity. Sitting in a hot tub next to water jets that massage and knead sore muscles and tender areas of the body, especially the lower back, is another example of hydrotherapy. So is sitting quietly in a sauna and cranking up the thermostat past 150 degrees Fahrenheit and allowing the damp heat to calm the body and slow down the activity of the internal organs.

Jordan, I learned while we were dating, was particularly excited about saunas. After asking me to marry him and presenting me with an engagement ring, he celebrated by buying "us" a portable home sauna. The sauna came in a kit, so after we married, Jordan set it up on our patio, and I fell in love with it too. Over seven years of marriage, I've used it hundreds of times. I like two things about our portable sauna: I can sit there and totally relax while I read a magazine, and I get so hot and sweaty that I *have* to drink several glasses of water to hydrate myself. I can feel my body sweating out the toxins.

**Jordan:** I love saunas and have become a fan and a proponent of hydrotherapy and water's healing properties. Water is nature's healer, a stress reducer that has favorable effects on skin and muscles. The most therapeutic forms of hydrotherapy involve hot *and* cold water. Hot water dilates blood vessels, which improves blood circulation, speeds the elimination of toxins, soothes sore muscles, opens clogged sinuses, and aids the endocrine system by stimulating nerve reflexes on the spinal cord. Cold water constricts blood vessels, numbs the nerves, slows respiration, and boosts oxygen use in the cells.

Nearly every time I take a shower, I alternate between blasts of hot water and cold water, which, I can assure you, is a dramatic way to stimulate local circulation. World-class athletes understand the importance of heat and cold. Meb Keflezighi, the Ethiopian-born distance runner who won the Olympic silver medal in the marathon for the United States at the Athens Games in 2004, finishes his twelve-mile training runs with quick dips in ice-cold mountain waters.[12]

*Back in the USSR*
*by Jordan Rubin*

I'm normally not a wild and crazy guy like Steve Martin, but I've performed a few wild and crazy stunts in my lifetime. One day after skiing my legs to a crisp on the slopes of Vail, Colorado, I talked Nicki into joining me in an outdoor hot tub under a blanket of stars. It felt invigorating to step out of my bath towel and into the freezing air before gently dunking my frame into steaming hot water.

That was the wild part. The crazy part was leaping out of the hot tub and flinging myself into a snow bank, where I flapped my arms and legs to make a snow angel. Talk about freezing!

**Nicki:** I stayed in the hot tub and couldn't believe what I was seeing. I wouldn't do what Jordan did for a million dollars. I can't stand to be freezing cold, and when he skedaddled back into the scalding water, he said it felt like a million pins were poking his skin. Not for me!

I think of that Rocky Mountain High every time I read a New Year's story about a "polar bear" club jumping into the freezing waters of Lake Michigan or Coney Island on January 1. But American dippers have nothing on the Russians, who step into Speedos and plunge into ice holes in the dead of winter—at midnight! It seems that every January 6, the feast of Epiphany, thousands of madcap Russians flock to frozen rivers and lakes to immerse themselves as a commemoration of the baptism of Christ. The temperature is usually well below zero.

I think I'll stick with snow angels.

But if you can't stand the thought of turning the cold nozzle way up in the shower, consider a cold footbath. Placing your feet in a tub filled to calf-depth cold water is an excellent alternative. But you don't have to go cold turkey, so to speak, with this hot shower/cold shower situation. Try cooling the water for fifteen or twenty seconds before raising the temperature almost to scalding. It's just a matter of getting used to it a few times. President Thomas Jefferson soaked his feet in cold water every morning for different reasons; he claimed that he didn't get colds by following this unusual practice.[13]

Another body therapy is adding several drops of essential oils to a drawn bath. Lavender, bergamot, cedarwood, chamomile, rosemary, and frankincense are wonderful scents that rise with the steam of the water. Taking a deep breath will soothe the mind and invigorate the spirit.

Essential oils are liquids that are generally distilled from leaves, stems, flowers, bark, roots, or other elements of a plant. Ancient civilizations in Israel, Egypt, India, Greece, and Rome relied on essential oils as the primary source of perfumes. In his work, Hippocrates, the father of medicine, described aromatic plant essences and the benefits of oil massage for its healing and mood-enhancing qualities.[14]

In the modern era, essential oils are used in the manufacture of high-quality perfumes. Don't let the word *oil* throw you off; there's nothing oily-feeling when an eyedropper of patchouli or lemongrass is mixed with hot bathwater. Essential oils are highly concentrated, but their fragrance has staying power.

Essential oils are a form of aromatherapy, and I like to take a couple of drops of lavender into the palms of my hands, rub them together, and then cup my hands as I lean over and breathe in the vapors. I often finish my advanced hygiene protocol with this action.

"The nose is a powerful sense organ, and the sense of smell is connected directly to the limbic system of the brain, which helps control emotions, memory, and several functions in the body," says the *Gale Encyclopedia of Alternative Medicine.* "Research has shown that aromas and the sense of smell influence memory recall, moods, and bodily responses such as heart rate, respiration, hormone levels, and stress reactions."[15]

Stimulate the nose with essential oils. You'll be surprised at the results.

## Let the Sunshine In

**Nicki:** Another form of body therapy, believe it or not, is sunbathing. When I was growing up, I loved summer, lying next to the pool in my swimsuit and getting a great tan. But like you, I've heard for years that you can get skin cancer from being out in the sun too much. *Melanoma* is a scary word, so whenever I've taken Joshua to the beach, I've slathered him with oily creams with a sun protection factor (SPF) of 30, lest he burn his baby skin.

But then Jordan asked an interesting question: "Why are we experiencing higher rates of skin cancer today when we spend 90 percent of our time indoors?"

I hadn't thought of that. Jordan also pointed out that our ancestors—who toiled outside from sunup to sundown—didn't get skin cancer at nearly the same rates as today. When I asked him why, he answered that he believes it's because we lack adequate nutrients in our diets and don't eat enough antioxidant-rich fruits, vegetables, and healthy fats, which naturally protect us from skin cancer.

**Jordan:** Contrary to conventional wisdom, sunbathing—or getting some sun during the day—is actually very healthy for you. Even though we've all heard about the dangers of developing skin cancer from lying on a blanket at the beach, the truth of the matter is that we need more sun, not less. Why? Because the body derives vitamin D—which keeps bones healthy and wards off cancer—from the sun. Physiologically speaking, the ultraviolet rays of sunlight warm the skin, which miraculously synthesizes vitamin D in ways extremely important to our bodies. Vitamin D plays a vital role in immunity and blood cell formation, and it has other cancer-fighting properties, as I mentioned in Key #2 when I talked about omega-3 cod-liver oil.

I'm pleased that the mainstream media are seeing the light, so to speak, and are agreeing with me. "Are Americans Dying from a Lack of Vitamin D?" asked a *Newsweek* article in 2005.[16] "Making a Case for Sun's Benefits," read a *Los Angeles Times* headline. The latter story, which called vitamin D the "sunshine vitamin," pointed toward studies suggesting that vitamin D was responsible for reducing the risk of lymphoma, improving the survival rate of lung cancer, and contributing to the decline of skin cancer, which the writer found "ironic."[17]

Not me. I didn't raise an eyebrow when I read that Dr. Edward Giovannucci, a Harvard University professor of medicine and nutrition, announced at a recent American Association for Cancer Research meeting that his research suggests that vitamin D from sunlight might prevent thirty deaths for each one caused by the sun.[18]

I urge you to incorporate sunbathing into your daily routine. I'm not talking about going off the deep end and lathering yourself up with Hawaiian Tropic tanning lotion while sunning yourself all afternoon. The National Institutes of Health (NIH) states that all you need is ten to fifteen minutes of sunlight for vitamin D synthesis to occur.

What you *don't* need to do is visit a tanning salon. I know that tanning salons are popular with women who want to keep that tan all year long, especially those who live in cold-weather climates and want to avoid the Casper-the-friendly-ghost look. I understand the rationale behind getting a good tan. Men and women look healthier, more attractive with a tan.

Those in the industry say that tanning booths are less dangerous than the sun, but the truth is, ultraviolet rays emitted from UV light sources in tanning salons are two to three times more powerful than the ultraviolet rays that occur naturally in the sun.[19] As with food, anything artificial is bad for you, and anything that God created—like sunlight—is good for you.

**Nicki:** I wish I had known that back in high school. I'll never forget the first time I used a tanning bed: I was a junior in high school, and prom was coming up. I visited a tanning salon a half dozen times before the big dance and got a great tan, but even back then I kept thinking that something didn't feel right about lying on a bed while an artificial light darkened my skin.

When I journeyed to Morehead State for my freshman year, the first thing I noticed was that everyone on campus had a tan—even the guys. When I joined a sorority, I felt the pressure to keep a tan face and body, so I purchased a package deal at a tanning salon that catered to Morehead State students.

I became a regular tanner. You could say that I was hooked by the look. I kept tanning for the next four or five years, even after I moved to the Sunshine State. A funny thing happened when I went to beach: after sunning myself for twenty minutes, I noticed the appearance of moles and sun spots on my arms and chest, and something told me that they were caused from years of using tanning beds. I haven't been back to a tanning palace since Jordan and I became serious, but I still have a ton of moles that weren't there before. If you're a tanning bed regular like I was, I urge you to stop now because they really aren't healthy for you.

**Jordan:** Exposing yourself to at least fifteen minutes of sunlight a day is necessary to increase vitamin D levels in your body. If you go outside to sun yourself, also consider practicing some deep-breathing exercises to eliminate toxins through the lungs. Start by inhaling slowly through the nose, which allows a deep breath of air to completely fill your lungs. Count to five as you breathe in, and then hold your breath for several seconds before exhaling through your mouth for several seconds. This allows oxygen to move quickly through your bloodstream.

Deep-breathing techniques are more involved than this simple description, but they are a peaceful, powerful tool to calm you down from the rigors of life while also restoring your energy. Taking a few minutes to practice deep-breathing exercises will soothe your mind and invigorate your spirit.

Moms in particular must reserve some energy to cope with the challenges of raising children, much like a good military general maintains a reserve force that can relieve exhausted soldiers who falter on the front lines. Practicing deep-breathing exercises, relaxing in the sun, and enjoying your favorite form of hydrotherapy will rejuvenate you.

**Nicki:** Another calming activity is music therapy, and the prescription is a simple one—listening to Christian praise and worship music. We love listening to Hillsong praise and worship songs. I love listening to a group called Third Day, but Casting Crowns, Jeremy Camp, and MercyMe rank right up there in my book. Jordan enjoys music by Stephen Curtis Chapman, his all-time favorite gospel artist.

The benefits of soothing music therapy have been known for centuries. Consider this Scripture from 1 Samuel 16:14–23 (NKJV):

> But the Spirit of the LORD departed from Saul, and a distressing spirit . . . troubled him. And Saul's servants said to him, "Surely, a distressing spirit . . . is troubling you. Let our master now command your servants . . . to seek out a man who is a skillful player on the harp. And it shall be that he will play it with his hand when the distressing spirit . . . is upon you, and you shall be well."
>
> So Saul said to his servants, "Provide me now a man who can play well, and bring him to me."
>
> Then one of the servants . . . said, "Look, I have seen a son of Jesse the Bethlehemite, who is skillful in playing . . . and the LORD is with him."
>
> Therefore Saul sent messengers to Jesse, and said, "Send me your son David, who is with the sheep." And Jesse took a donkey loaded with bread, a skin of wine, and a young goat, and sent them by his son David to Saul. So David came to Saul and stood before him. And he loved him greatly, and he became his armorbearer. Then Saul sent to Jesse, saying, "Please let David stand before me, for he has found favor in my sight." And so it was, whenever

> the [distressing spirit] . . . was upon Saul, that David would take a harp and play it with his hand. Then Saul would become refreshed and well, and the distressing spirit would depart from him.

As this story demonstrates, music therapy promotes relaxation, refreshment, and healing. Sometimes when Joshua was fussy as an infant, I would pick him up in my arms and walk him and sing to him. One of the songs I would sing was the praise song "Thy Word," written by Michael W. Smith.

It worked nearly every time.

*What Women Are Saying*
*by Doris Bailey*

When I was just fifteen, I was a young woman trying to find her place in a big world but acutely aware of rejection and not having any friends. I was diminutive in stature—just five feet, two inches tall—but carrying too much weight at 185 pounds. At school, I preferred to remain in the background, where I wouldn't be noticed—or rejected.

One evening my older brother, Sonny, a senior in high school, invited some of his buddies to hang out. The boys were cutting up and joking around when one of them caught my eye.

"Hey, Doris, want an apple?" he asked. He reached for a shiny Red Delicious stacked in a bowl of fruit on the dining room table.

"Sure," I responded, not giving the question a second thought.

The boy tossed the apple underhand across the room, which I caught. I had just sunk my teeth in the sweet apple when he suddenly belted out, "Hey everybody, look at the pig!"

All the guys turned toward me as I froze in mid-bite, which only accentuated the image of a pig roasting on a spit with an apple in its mouth. Laughter erupted, which mortified me. I ran for my bedroom, where I fell on my bed and bawled my eyes out the rest of the evening.

What that boy said that night has stuck with me all my life. I never had a good feeling about myself before that night, and I certainly didn't think very highly of myself after that.

I gained weight steadily after I married because I loved going to Perry Boy's, an all-you-can-eat restaurant, and filling up my plate with ham, bacon, fried chicken, mashed potatoes, and corn, making five or six trips through the buffet line. My weight slowly but surely marched past 280 pounds after my second son, Brian, was born.

After twelve years of marriage, Jack and I divorced. I moved to Central California and settled in Modesto, where I met and married Larry Bailey in 1982 while working as a certified nursing assistant in nursing and private homes. When my weight crept north of 300 pounds, I gave up hope of ever slimming down. I tried the popular diets: Overeater's Anonymous, Jenny Craig, and Weight Watchers, but they never worked. I would lose five pounds, but then I would overeat a little bit or not follow the diet to a T and get six pounds back. That was really frustrating.

Then, on a Sunday morning, I heard Jordan Rubin speak at our church about presenting our bodies as living sacrifices. He challenged us that morning. "Can you say, 'This is the best I have, and I'm giving it to the Lord'?" he asked. "Are you an example of God's best? Wouldn't it be awesome if God's people were so full of good health, so vibrant, that others would notice us from ten or twenty feet away?"

I didn't want to be noticed. Decades of obesity had taken their toll: asthma, gout, osteoarthritis, acid reflux, high blood pressure, and sleep apnea. My knees were shot: the only way I could walk was with the assistance of a cane or walker.

I went home and cleaned out my cupboards and refrigerator, and then I went shopping for foods that God created. I began eating many more salads and either baked or broiled chicken. I stopped eating pork and sugary treats like jelly-filled doughnuts and apple turnovers. No more eating a half-gallon of ice cream in one sitting. I filled my refrigerator with fresh vegetables, organic whole milk, and even some goat's milk and goat's cheese, though

I wasn't too hip on that in the beginning. I ate apples, bananas, or oranges as my lunch.

I saw pounds immediately come off—and stay off. What a blessing for someone who had tried every diet for the last thirty-eight years with no sustained weight loss or health improvement until I tried the Great Physician's prescription. In a couple of months, I lost twenty-five pounds, going from 330 to 305 pounds.

I'm encouraged to keep following what I have learned, and now I have given myself a new goal: to get down to 175 pounds within two years!

## Rx THE GREAT PHYSICIAN'S RX FOR WOMEN'S HEALTH: CONDITION YOUR BODY WITH EXERCISE AND BODY THERAPIES

- *Go to sleep earlier, paying close attention to how much sleep you get before midnight. Do your best to get eight hours of sleep nightly. Remember that sleep is the most important nonnutrient you can incorporate into your health regimen.*
- *Make a commitment to exercise three times a week or more.*
- *Incorporate five to fifteen minutes of functional fitness into your daily schedule.*
- *End your next shower by changing the water temperature to cool (or cold) and standing underneath the spray for one minute.*
- *Integrate essential oils into your daily life.*

- *Take a brisk walk and see how much better you feel at the end of the day.*
- *Make a conscious effort to practice deep-breathing exercises once a day. Inflate your lungs to full and hold for several seconds before slowly exhaling.*
- *Play worship music in your home, in your car, or on your iPod. Focus on God's plan for your life.*

## THE GREAT PHYSICIAN'S RX FOR WEEK #4

Remember to visit www.BiblicalHealthInstitute.com and click on the GPRx Resource Guide to learn more about the foods and nutritional supplements recommended in the Great Physician's Rx 7 Weeks of Wellness plan. You can also find more than 250 healthy and delicious recipes, including the italicized recipes in this chapter, at this site.

### DAY 22

*You will notice that some items in the meal plans that follow are italicized. You can find the recipes for these—and over other 250 delicious and healthy recipes—at www.BiblicalHealthInstitute.com.*

***Upon Waking***

*Advanced hygiene:* By now you have read Key #3 on practicing advanced hygiene, and you have used these methods for several days in your morning routine. You will continue to use what you've learned, but I won't spell it out in detail in this chapter. The note will just say, "Practice advanced hygiene." If you need a refresher on the directions, please see "A Refresher on Practicing Advanced Hygiene," following Key #7 on page 277.

*Supplements*: Take one serving of a fiber/green superfood combination containing ground flaxseed, mixed in 12 to 16 ounces of water or raw vegetable juice.

*Exercise:* Perform functional fitness exercises for five minutes, similar to those described in this chapter. During exercise, drink 8 ounces of water.

***Breakfast***

During breakfast, drink 8 ounces of water.

two eggs (omega-3 or organic, and prepared as desired)

one piece of fruit

one piece of whole-grain sprouted or sourdough toast with butter

hot tea with honey

*Supplements:* Take two whole food multivitamin caplets, one capsule of omega-3 cod-liver oil, and two caplets of a whole food calcium/magnesium blend.

***Between Breakfast and Lunch***

Drink 12 ounces of water.

***Lunch***

During lunch, drink 8 ounces of water.

green salad with 3 ounces of chicken and carrots, red onions, cucumbers, and yellow peppers

healthy salad dressing with one tablespoon of extra-virgin olive oil or high-lignan flaxseed oil

one piece of fruit

*Supplements:* Take two whole food multivitamin caplets, one capsule of omega-3 cod-liver oil, and two caplets of a whole food calcium/magnesium blend.

***Between Lunch and Dinner***

Drink 12 ounces of water.

***Dinner***

During dinner, drink 8 ounces of water.

fish of choice

brown rice

green salad with red or yellow peppers, red onions, green or red cabbage, celery, cucumbers, and carrots

healthy salad dressing with olive oil and/or high-lignan flaxseed oil

*Supplements:* Take two whole food multivitamin caplets, one capsule of omega-3 cod-liver oil, and two caplets of a whole food calcium/magnesium blend.

***Snack/Dessert***

apple cinnamon whole food bar (with beta-glucans from soluble oat fiber)

whole-milk yogurt, fruit, and honey

***Before Bed***

*Exercise:* Go for a walk outdoors.

*Supplements:* Take one serving of a fiber/green superfood combination containing ground flaxseed, mixed in 12 to 16 ounces of water or raw vegetable juice.

*Advanced hygiene:* Practice advanced hygiene.

## DAY 23

*You will notice that some items in the meal plans that follow are italicized. You can find the recipes for these—and over other 250 delicious and healthy recipes—at www.BiblicalHealthInstitute.com.*

***Upon Waking***

*Advanced hygiene:* Practice advanced hygiene.

*Supplements:* Take one serving of a fiber/green superfood combination containing ground flaxseed, mixed in 12 to 16 ounces of water or raw vegetable juice.

*Exercise:* Perform functional fitness exercises for five minutes, and do deep-breathing exercises for five minutes. During exercise, drink 8 ounces of water.

*Body therapy:* Take a hot-and-cold shower. After a normal shower, alternate sixty seconds of water as hot as you can stand it, followed by sixty seconds of water as cold as you can stand it. Repeat cycle twice for a total of four minutes, finishing with cold.

*Breakfast*

During breakfast, drink 8 ounces of water.

For a healthy smoothie, mix the following in a blender:

8 ounces plain whole milk, yogurt, or kefir

1 tablespoon honey

1/2 cup fresh or frozen fruit (bananas, peaches, berries, pineapple, etc.)

1 teaspoon high-lignan flaxseed oil

1 serving of protein powder (optional)

*Supplements:* Take two whole food multivitamin caplets, one capsule of omega-3 cod-liver oil, and two caplets of a whole food calcium/magnesium blend.

*Between Breakfast and Lunch*

Drink 12 ounces of water.

*Lunch*

During lunch, drink 8 ounces of water.

low-mercury, high omega-3 tuna on sprouted or yeast-free whole-grain bread, with lettuce, tomato, and sprouts

one piece of fruit

*Supplements:* Take two whole food multivitamin caplets, one capsule of omega-3 cod-liver oil, and two caplets of a whole food calcium/magnesium blend.

*Between Lunch and Dinner*

Drink 12 ounces of water.

*Dinner*

During dinner, drink 8 ounces of water.

chicken dish of choice

millet with onions, mushrooms, and peas

*Supplements:* Take two whole food multivitamin caplets, one capsule of omega-3 cod-liver oil, and two caplets of a whole food calcium/magnesium blend.

***Snack/Dessert***

whole food meal replacement powder (with beta-glucans from soluble oat fiber) mixed in 12 ounces of water

cottage cheese, honey, and berries

***Before Bed***

*Exercise:* Go for a short walk outdoors.

*Supplements:* Take one serving of a fiber/green superfood combination containing ground flaxseed, mixed in 12 to 16 ounces of water or raw vegetable juice.

*Advanced hygiene:* Practice advanced hygiene.

*Body therapy:* Spend ten minutes listening to soothing music before you retire.

## DAY 24

*You will notice that some items in the meal plans that follow are italicized. You can find the recipes for these—and over other 250 delicious and healthy recipes—at www.BiblicalHealthInstitute.com.*

***Upon Waking***

*Advanced hygiene:* Practice advanced hygiene.

*Supplements:* Take one serving of a fiber/green superfood combination containing ground flaxseed, mixed in 12 to 16 ounces of water or raw vegetable juice.

*Exercise:* Perform functional fitness exercises for five minutes, or spend ten minutes on a minitrampoline (also known as a rebounder). Finish with five minutes of deep-breathing exercises. During exercise, drink 8 ounces of water.

*Body therapy:* Get twenty minutes of direct sunlight.

***Breakfast***

During breakfast, drink 8 ounces of water.

*Five-Grain Porridge* with two tablespoons of protein powder added after cooking strawberries

hot tea with honey

*Supplements:* Take two whole food multivitamin caplets, one capsule of omega-3 cod-liver oil, and two caplets of a whole food calcium/magnesium blend.

***Between Breakfast and Lunch***

Drink 12 ounces of water.

***Lunch***

During lunch, drink 8 ounces of water.

green salad with 3 ounces of steak and carrots, red onions, cucumbers, and yellow peppers

healthy salad dressing with one tablespoon of extra-virgin olive oil or high-lignan flaxseed oil

one piece of fruit

*Supplements:* Take two whole food multivitamin caplets, one capsule of omega-3 cod-liver oil, and two caplets of a whole food calcium/magnesium blend.

***Between Lunch and Dinner***

Drink 12 ounces of water.

***Dinner***

During dinner, drink 8 ounces of water.

red meat of choice

baked sweet potato with butter

green salad with red or yellow peppers, red onions, green or red cabbage, celery, cucumbers, and carrots

healthy salad dressing with olive oil and/or high-lignan flaxseed oil

*Supplements:* Take two whole food multivitamin caplets, one capsule of omega-3 cod-liver oil, and two caplets of a whole food calcium/magnesium blend.

***Snack/Dessert***

berry antioxidant whole food bar (with beta-glucans from soluble oat fiber)

apple and almond or sesame butter (tahini)

***Before Bed***

*Exercise:* Go for a walk outdoors or participate in a favorite sport or recreational activity.

*Supplements:* Take one serving of a fiber/green superfood combination containing ground flaxseed, mixed in 12 to 16 ounces of water or raw vegetable juice.

*Body therapy:* Take a warm bath for fifteen minutes, with one cup of Epsom salt added.

*Advanced hygiene:* Practice advanced hygiene.

*Sleep:* Go to bed by 11:30 p.m.

## DAY 25

*You will notice that some items in the meal plans that follow are italicized. You can find the recipes for these—and over other 250 delicious and healthy recipes—at www.BiblicalHealthInstitute.com.*

***Upon Waking***

*Advanced hygiene:* Practice advanced hygiene.

*Supplements:* Take one serving of a fiber/green superfood combination containing ground flaxseed, mixed in 12 to 16 ounces of water or raw vegetable juice.

*Exercise:* Perform functional fitness exercises for fifteen minutes, or spend fifteen minutes on the rebounder. Finish with five minutes of deep-breathing exercises. During exercise, drink 8 ounces of water.

*Body therapy:* Take a hot-and-cold shower: After a normal shower, alternate sixty seconds of water as hot as you can stand it, followed by sixty seconds of water as cold as you can stand it. Repeat cycle three times for a total of six minutes, finishing with cold.

***Breakfast***

During breakfast, drink 8 ounces of water.

For a healthy smoothie, mix the following in a blender:

8 ounces plain whole milk, yogurt, or kefir

1 tablespoon honey

1/2 cup fresh or frozen fruit (bananas, peaches, berries, pineapple, etc.)

1 teaspoon high-lignan flaxseed oil

1 serving of protein powder (optional)

*Supplements:* Take two whole food multivitamin caplets, one capsule of omega-3 cod-liver oil, and two caplets of a whole food calcium/magnesium blend.

***Between Breakfast and Lunch***

Drink 12 ounces of water.

***Lunch***

During lunch, drink 8 ounces of water.

turkey on sprouted or yeast-free whole-grain bread with lettuce, tomato, and sprouts

one piece of fruit

*Supplements:* Take two whole food multivitamin caplets, one capsule of omega-3 cod-liver oil, and two caplets of a whole food calcium/magnesium blend.

***Between Lunch and Dinner***

Drink 12 ounces of water.

***Dinner***

During dinner, drink 8 ounces of water.

*Salmon Lemon Sauté*

steamed asparagus

green salad with red or yellow peppers, red onions, green or red cabbage, celery, cucumbers, and carrots

healthy salad dressing with olive oil and/or high-lignan flaxseed oil

*Supplements:* Take two whole food multivitamin caplets, one capsule of omega-3 cod-liver oil, and two caplets of a whole food calcium/magnesium blend.

***Snack/Dessert***

whole food meal replacement powder (with beta-glucans from soluble oat fiber) mixed in 12 ounces of water

flax crackers, whole grain crackers, or baked corn chips and hummus, salsa, or guacamole

***Before Bed***

*Exercise:* Go for a walk outdoors or participate in a favorite sport or recreational activity.

*Supplements:* Take one serving of a fiber/green superfood combination containing ground flaxseed, mixed in 12 to 16 ounces of water or raw vegetable juice.

*Advanced hygiene:* Practice advanced hygiene.

*Body therapy:* Spend ten minutes listening to soothing music before you retire.

*Sleep:* Go to bed by 11:15 p.m.

## DAY 26 (PARTIAL-FAST DAY)

*You will notice that some items in the meal plans that follow are italicized. You can find the recipes for these—and over other 250 delicious and healthy recipes—at www.BiblicalHealthInstitute.com.*

***Upon Waking***

*Advanced hygiene:* Practice advanced hygiene.

*Supplements:* Take one serving of a fiber/green superfood combination containing ground flaxseed, mixed in 12 to 16 ounces of water or raw vegetable juice.

*Exercise:* Perform functional fitness exercises for fifteen minutes, or spend fifteen minutes on the rebounder. Finish with five minutes of deep-breathing exercises. During exercise, drink 8 ounces of water.

*Body therapy:* Get twenty minutes of direct sunlight.

***Breakfast***

none (partial-fast day)

Drink 12 ounces of water.

***Between Breakfast and Lunch***

Drink 12 ounces of water.

***Lunch***

none (partial-fast day)

Drink 12 ounces of water.

***Between Lunch and Dinner***

Drink 12 ounces of water.

***Dinner***

During dinner, drink 8 ounces of water.

*Chicken Soup*

cultured vegetables

green salad with red or yellow peppers, red onions, green or red cabbage, celery, cucumbers, and carrots

healthy salad dressing with olive oil and/or high-lignan flaxseed oil

*Supplements:* Take two whole food multivitamin caplets, one capsule of omega-3 cod-liver oil, and two caplets of a whole food calcium/magnesium blend.

***Snack/Dessert***

none (partial-fast day)

Drink 12 ounces of water.

***Before Bed***

*Exercise:* Go for a walk outdoors or participate in a favorite sport or recreational activity.

*Supplements:* Take one serving of a fiber/green superfood combination containing ground flaxseed, mixed in 12 to 16 ounces of water or raw vegetable juice.

*Body therapy:* Take a warm bath, with eight drops of biblical essential oils added, for fifteen minutes.

*Advanced hygiene:* Practice advanced hygiene.

*Sleep:* Go to bed by 11:00 p.m.

## DAY 27 (DAY OF REST)

*You will notice that some items in the meal plans that follow are italicized. You can find the recipes for these—and over other 250 delicious and healthy recipes—at www.BiblicalHealthInstitute.com.*

### *Upon Waking*

*Advanced hygiene:* Practice advanced hygiene. See page 277 for guidance.

*Supplements:* Take one serving of a fiber/green superfood combination containing ground flaxseed, mixed in 12 to 16 ounces of water or raw vegetable juice.

*Exercise:* Do no formal exercise since it's a day of rest.

*Body therapies:* None.

### *Breakfast*

During breakfast, drink 8 ounces of water.

one whole-grain pancake with maple syrup and butter

4 ounces of whole-milk yogurt with berries and honey and 1/2 teaspoon of high-lignan flaxseed oil (optional)

organic fresh-ground coffee with organic cream and honey

*Supplements:* Take two whole food multivitamin caplets, one capsule of omega-3 cod-liver oil, and two caplets of a whole food calcium/magnesium blend.

### *Between Breakfast and Lunch*

Drink 12 ounces of water.

### *Lunch*

During lunch, drink 8 ounces of water.

green salad with raw cheese, avocado, walnuts, olives, carrots, red onions, cucumbers, and yellow peppers

healthy salad dressing with one tablespoon of extra-virgin olive oil or high-lignan flaxseed oil

one piece of fruit

Supplements: Take two whole food multivitamin caplets, one capsule of omega-3 cod-liver oil, and two caplets of a whole food calcium/magnesium blend.

***Between Lunch and Dinner***

Drink 12 ounces of water.

***Dinner***

During dinner, drink 8 ounces of water.

grilled wild salmon

quinoa with onions and mushrooms

Italian-style zucchini

*Supplements:* Take two whole food multivitamin caplets, one capsule of omega-3 cod-liver oil, and two caplets of a whole food calcium/magnesium blend.

***Snack/Dessert***

green superfood whole food bar (with beta-glucans from soluble oat fiber)

raw nuts, seeds, and dried fruit

***Before Bed***

*Exercise:* None.

*Body therapies:* None.

*Supplements:* Take one serving of a fiber/green superfood combination containing ground flaxseed, mixed in 12 to 16 ounces of water or raw vegetable juice.

*Advanced hygiene*: Practice advanced hygiene.

*Sleep:* Go to bed by 11:00 p.m.

## Day 28

*You will notice that some items in the meal plans that follow are italicized. You can find the recipes for these—and over other 250 delicious and healthy recipes—at www.BiblicalHealthInstitute.com.*

*Upon Waking*

*Advanced hygiene:* Practice advanced hygiene.

*Supplements:* Take one serving of a fiber/green superfood combination containing ground flaxseed, mixed in 12 to 16 ounces of water or raw vegetable juice.

*Exercise:* Perform functional fitness exercises for fifteen minutes, or spend fifteen minutes on the rebounder. Finish with five minutes of deep-breathing exercises. During exercise, drink 8 ounces of water.

*Body therapy:* Take a hot-and-cold shower, following directions from previous days.

*Breakfast*

During breakfast, drink 8 ounces of water.

two-egg omelet with avocado, cheese, tomato, onion, and pepper

*Sautéed Veggies*

hot tea and honey

*Supplements:* Take two whole food multivitamin caplets, one capsule of omega-3 cod-liver oil, and two caplets of a whole food calcium/magnesium blend.

*Between Breakfast and Lunch*

Drink 12 ounces of water.

*Lunch*

During lunch, drink 8 ounces of water.

almond butter and honey or pure fruit jam on sprouted or yeast-free whole-grain bread

one piece of fruit

*Supplements:* Take two whole food multivitamin caplets, one capsule of omega-3 cod-liver oil, and two caplets of a whole food calcium/magnesium blend.

*Between Lunch and Dinner*

Drink 12 ounces of water.

***Dinner***

During dinner, drink 8 ounces of water.

chicken dish of choice

green salad with red or yellow peppers, red onions, green or red cabbage, celery, cucumbers, and carrots

healthy salad dressing with olive oil and/or high-lignan flaxseed oil

*Supplements:* Take two whole food multivitamin caplets, one capsule of omega-3 cod-liver oil, and two caplets of a whole food calcium/magnesium blend.

***Snack/Dessert***

whole food meal replacement powder (with beta-glucans from soluble oat fiber) mixed in 12 ounces of water

*Quick Sprouted Apple Crisp*

***Before Bed***

*Exercise:* Go for a walk outdoors or participate in a favorite sport or recreational activity.

*Supplements:* Take one serving of a fiber/green superfood combination containing ground flaxseed, mixed in 12 to 16 ounces of water or raw vegetable juice.

*Advanced hygiene:* Practice advanced hygiene.

*Body therapy:* Spend ten minutes listening to soothing music before you retire.

*Sleep:* Go to bed by 10:30 p.m.

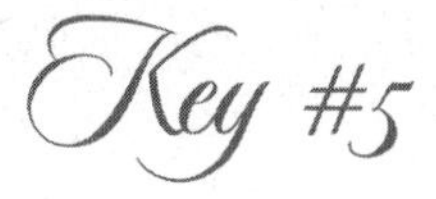

# Key #5

## *Reduce Toxins in Your Environment*

**Nicki:** When Joshua was fourteen months old, we decided to put him in swimming lessons. There was a pool nearby, so we enrolled him to teach him the fundamentals of staying afloat.

But after the second or third session, I noticed something different about Joshua. He acted as though his stomach hurt. Even worse, he had the worst poopy diapers I had ever encountered. I talked to my girlfriends about this, and they said, "Oh, if he's going in a chlorine pool, then he's going to have messy diapers and a stomachache afterward." Sure enough, each time he took a swimming lesson, it wasn't long before he had both.

**Jordan:** Joshua's story is a reminder that we're living in a toxic world that includes swimming pools brimming with chlorinated water. I'm passionate about this issue because I'm very concerned with environmental toxins and how they can poison our bodies because of our around-the-clock exposure to numerous chemical concentrations, both minute and large. Toxins enter our bodies through the air we breathe, the water we drink, the foods we eat, the things we touch, the products we apply to our skin, and even the pools we swim in. This chemical residue is referred to as a person's *body burden*, a chemical legacy that scientists say is the result of decades of our increasing reliance on synthetic chemicals in our everyday lives. It's becoming more evident that while advances in chemistry have made life more comfortable, we all could be paying a heavy price tomorrow and beyond.

Whether or not you're aware of it—and I'd say that very few people are—hundreds, if not thousands, of chemical compounds taint our food, our homes, our bloodstreams, and ultimately our children. You have to ask yourself why autism, which used to afflict one in 10,000 children, is now the scourge of one in 166 kids today? Why have childhood asthma rates exploded?[1] Closer to home, Nicki had great difficulty in becoming pregnant, as do millions of couples. (One in twelve American couples of reproductive age are infertile.[2]) Was her bout with infertility related to a lifelong exposure to environmental pollutants and chemicals?

I think about that every now and then, and recently our public health officials have given more thought and research to the significance of toxins in our environment. The Centers for Disease Control and Prevention has released three assessments of the nation's collective body burden since 1999, and each "biomonitoring" report shows how we're becoming more and more contaminated from a stew of pesticides, solvents, plastics, and metals that are the result of living in a material world. The latest report, issued in 2005, declared that CDC scientists looked for 148 environmental chemicals in blood and urine samples from a random sample of several thousand participants. As a way of comparison, the initial report in 1999 tested for only 27,[3] yet nearly 80,000 chemicals are registered for use in commerce today.

The major findings in 2005 were that children have higher concentrations of stored chemicals than adults, especially heavy metals, pesticides, and a family of chemicals called *phthalates*, which are used to increase plastic's flexibility and resiliency. Women of childbearing age continue to show a high exposure to mercury, which is harmful to an unborn baby growing in the womb. "We have fouled our own nest," said pediatrician Jerry Paulson, MD, a spokesman for Physicians for Social Responsibility, following the release of the *Third National Report on Human Exposure to Environmental Chemicals*. "We've contaminated the environment sufficiently that there are measurable amounts of potentially toxic substances in people—kids and adults."[4]

The body attempts to absorb and excrete toxins in different ways. Water-soluble toxins, things like uric acid and ammonia, are primarily excreted in urine, while others, like carbon dioxide and benzodiazepines, are released from the skin and lungs. Fat-soluble chemicals, such as dioxins, phthalates, and chlorine, accumulate in our fatty tissues, where they may persist for months or years before they're eliminated from our systems, mainly through our bowels and perspiration. Though it would be impossible to go back to a pristine, Garden of Eden–like world, it behooves us to take steps to protect ourselves and our children from the potentially harmful toxins in our environment, which is the fifth key to unlocking your health potential.

### *Estrogen Dominance, Part II*
### *by Pancheta Wilson, MD*

In Key #2, the chapter dealing with the importance of adding nutritional supplements to your diet, I described how an imbalance of estrogen, the female hormone, leads to a wide range of illnesses, including an exacerbation of endometriosis, *Candida albicans,* and insomnia. This hormonal imbalance was studied for years by Harvard-trained John Lee, MD, the physician who coined the term "estrogen dominance." Hormonal imbalance is created when the ratio of estrogen to progesterone sways too much in one direction—usually in the direction of excess estrogen, which, in turn, "dominates" the body. Dr. Lee declared that millions of women are suffering from a relative lack of progesterone compared to estrogen in their bodies.

Estrogen imbalance is caused by several factors. Levels of estrogen naturally reduce between the ages of thirty-five and fifty, the perimenopausal years that are part of the aging process. Birth control pills, which contain estrogen, and estrogen-replacement therapy (ERT) contribute to a worsening of estrogen dominance, but the biggest contributor to estrogen dominance may be related to environmental factors.

Estrogenlike hormones and chemicals are found in certain foods that we eat. It's no secret that much of our nation's livestock are fed with grain, hay, and feed containing nitrates and antibiotics. Some animals are fed with pesticide-treated feed and grass. This is why I advocate eating organic and pasture-fed meat.

Much of the cattle in the U.S. routinely chew on feed with hormones such as *melengestrol acetate,* or MGA, which improves the growth rate in feedlot heifers, and buffers containing sodium bicarbonate, which naturalizes the acidity in the digestive tract. These additives help livestock owners fatten up their herds, which, in turn, fattens their bottom lines. These practices, however, pass along a myriad of hormone-disrupting toxins to those who dine on these meats.

The fatty tissues of farm-raised fish are magnets for a host of toxins received from eating pellets of ground-up fish meat. They range from polychlorinated biphenyls (PCBs), a group of chemicals used in paint, ink, and dye, to dioxins and metals present in the environment. Mercury, a heavy metal, is especially prevalent in some canned tuna. Pesticide residue generally coats conventionally grown fruits and vegetables, and petrochemical compounds found in household toiletries—soap, shampoo, and conditioners—often have chemical structures similar to estrogen and can therefore add to the effect of this hormone.

One would have to live in a bubble to escape the excess estrogenlike compounds that we're exposed to from the chemicals contained in creams, lotion, hairspray, and room deodorizers as well as industrial solvents used to clean our floors, kitchens, and bathrooms. I encourage concerned women to take a saliva test to identify whether or not you have an estrogen imbalance. A clinical laboratory can test for the following eight hormones: estradiol, estrone, estriol, progesterone, testosterone, DHEAs, androstenedione, and cortisol. (Ask your doctor about saliva testing or learn more about an in-home test at www.salivatest.com. Dr. Joseph Mercola recommends Aeron Labs at 1-800-631-7900.)

Once you have results, you should consult with a licensed practitioner who specializes in hormone therapy. In my office, I support women who wish to get off hormone replacement therapy (HRT), such as Premarin, Provera, or PremPro, and a long list of others. According to Dr. Lee, those using HRT drugs have a 29 percent higher risk of breast cancer, a 26 percent higher risk of heart disease, and a 41 percent higher risk of stroke, not to mention side effects like weight gain, fatigue, depression, irritability, headaches, insomnia, bloating, low libido, gallbladder disease, and blood clots.[5]

I do recommend using natural hormone therapy, along with progesterone cream. There are effective plant-derived estrogens obtained from a wild yam grown in Mexico. Progesterone in cream has the identical chemical structure to that which is synthesized by the ovarian corpus luteum, and it is easily absorbed through the skin.

I have confidently instructed hundreds of perimenopausal and menopausal women over the years regarding the use of natural HRT. Though some report bouts of sleeplessness, many express relief that their symptoms have been relieved and that they feel like themselves again. Hot flashes are a distant memory.

I urge you to learn more about natural therapy-progesterone cream as well as bio-identical hormone therapy, which is created from isolated plant extracts and administered orally and in transdermal cream. These creams can increase vitality, renew emotional balance, and improve your skin.

## TOXIC ADDITIVES

**Jordan:** While most of the heavy metals inside the body are a result of environmental contamination due to industrial uses, it doesn't help matters when we eat foods laced with chemicals and fruits and vegetables doused with pesticides. Liz Lipski, PhD, author of *Digestive Wellness,* points out that the average American consumes fourteen pounds of additives a year.[6] Foods that God definitely did not create come with food colorings, preservatives, flavorings, emulsifiers, humectants, and antimicrobials.

In my opinion, among the worst additives are no-calorie and low-calorie artificial sweeteners such as these:

- the blue packets of Equal, which contain aspartame
- the pink packets of Sweet'N Low, which contain saccharin
- the yellow packets of Splenda, which contain sucralose

These chemicals are several hundred times—if not thousands—sweeter than sugar and found in every sit-down restaurant in America. An upstart named Sunett, made from Acesulfame K, is trying to earn a seat at the table, as is Aclame, which is 2,000 times sweeter than sucrose. They are looking for a long sip from a huge market: as many as 180 million Americans regularly eat and drink sugar-free products, according to recent statistics by the Calorie Control Council.[7] But how toxic are artificial sweeteners?

Well, I have a colleague whose grandmother hung out a hummingbird feeder in the backyard, filling it with sugared water to attract hummingbirds. One time, she ran out of sugar, so she mixed Splenda with some water. The next day, to her horror, she discovered three dead hummingbirds in her yard.

Okay, so you're not going to fall from the sky like a dead hummingbird if someone spikes your iced tea with Splenda, but in the court of scientific opinion, artificial sweeteners have been the subject of intense debate and research for the last forty years, ever since cyclamate—a no-calorie sweetener used in diet soft drinks like Tab—was banned by the Food and Drug Administration in 1970.

Diet sodas have no nutritional value, so drinking a diet drink with artificial sweeteners is a nonstarter in my book anyway. Besides the long-alleged cancer risks, sugar alcohols and polyols such as sorbitol, malitol, isomalt, and a whole lot of other scientific-sounding names found in popular artificial sweeteners can create significant digestive problems. Dr. Prabhakar Swaroop, assistant professor of gastroenterology at Saint Louis University, said, "These sugar alcohols are made up of long chains, and our bodies have a hard time breaking them down." In large amounts, they can cause diarrhea, gas, and bloating—what people refer to as a "laxative effect," he added.[8]

When it comes to the chemical health risks of conventionally produced foods, I recommend organic food, which, by definition, is food grown or produced without using pesticides, in Key #1. Now an additional environmental issue has surfaced in recent years: genetically modifying crops, such as soybeans, corn, cotton, and canola. They're called "GM foods" or "biotech" crops.

All living things have a genetic code in their cells that make them grow a certain way. Since the 1990s, scientists have discovered how to change the genes in plants to make them grow higher, larger, denser—and more resistant to insect infestation—but others fear that genetic engineering will unleash an environmental disaster on the public. Critics have called genetically modified crops "Frankenfood" or "agricultural asbestos," and I wouldn't knowingly eat a product made from a GM crop.

I don't think more than a handful of people are aware that almost a third of the agricultural land in the United States is planted with gene-altered crops,[9] even though 41 percent of Americans claimed they knew that GM foods were sold in grocery stores, according to Pew Research.[10] Many shoppers unwittingly fill their shopping carts with genetically modified foods because roughly 75 percent of processed foods—cooking oils, boxed cereals, grain products, and frozen dinners—contain some GM ingredients, according to the Grocery Manufacturers of America.[11] This news is another reason to only eat foods that God created, in a form healthy for the body.

If you are the person who usually does the food shopping for the home, I urge you to buy organic as far as your food budget will take you. As *Consumer Reports* magazine said, "A growing body of research shows that pesticides and other contaminants are more prevalent in the foods we eat than we thought. And studies show that by eating organic foods, you can reduce your exposure to potential health risks associated with these chemicals."[12]

In an interesting trend piece, the *Los Angeles Times Magazine* noted the start of a burgeoning movement called "sustainable food," which means the establishment of a shorter food chain by restaurants and consumers eager to buy meat, fruits, and vegetables produced locally. Currently, only 1 to 2 percent of America's food is locally grown, and the produce you eat is shipped an average of 1,500 miles to your local supermarket, according to a 2001 study by the Leopold Center for Sustainable Agriculture at Iowa State University.[13]

The leaders of the sustainable food movement urge consumers to seek out organic alternatives to mainstream food from co-ops, natural food stores, farmer's markets, roadside stands, and backyard gardens and fruit-bearing trees. As for the higher cost of buying local, proponents say that you can pay your farmer now, or you can pay your doctor later. Nothing truer was ever said about the virtues of eating organic.

*To Microwave or Not to Microwave?*
*by Nicki Rubin*

We don't have a microwave in our home.

For some women, that would be like saying, "You won't find a hair dryer in the bathroom." Ninety percent of American kitchens come equipped with a microwave oven to heat up leftovers or frozen meals. But while Jordan and I were setting up house after the honeymoon, he took one look at my microwave and shook his head. Microwave ovens, he said, emit radiation in the form of radio frequencies. When these waves of energy bombard food, the agitation causes molecular friction to occur, which destroys the fragile structure of vitamins, minerals, and enzymes in food.

The Food and Drug Administration (FDA) regulates microwave ovens and believes they are safe for use, but the jury is still out on the possibility of a link between microwave exposure and diseases such as cancer. We decided we'd rather not take any chances. Why risk it?

I haven't missed having a microwave, even after I stopped breastfeeding and needed to warm up formula. It only takes a couple more minutes to heat a pot of water and warm up his bottle. Nor have I missed "zapping" leftovers in a microwave. I've found that when I want to heat up something quick, an old-school toaster oven saves the day. I can cook lamb chops, baked potatoes, and just about any leftover in the fridge with a toaster oven. They heat up faster than regular ovens, use less energy, and are easier to clean.

My favorite toaster-oven meal is homemade pizzas made from sprouted English muffins, which are not only a healthy source of fiber and other nutrients, but heat up in a jiffy and don't have a soggy aftertaste as some microwaved foods do.

## Take a Deep Breath

**Jordan:** Another environmental issue looming large is the presence of airborne toxins in our homes. Regarding the air we breathe, double-pane windows and year-round heating and air conditioning ensure that fresh air stays outside, and stale, chemically tainted air dwells inside. Today's well-insulated homes and energy-efficient windows and doors trap "used" air with harmful particles of carbon dioxide, nitrogen dioxide, and pet dander. In office buildings, heating, cooling, and ventilation systems that are not properly maintained are frequent sources of airborne toxins such as asbestos and nitrogen dioxide.

Perhaps you've noticed all the attention given to mold-related illnesses and how homes have been torn up to rid walls and studs of spores of green and black mold. Those living in mold-infested environments have been diagnosed with impaired thyroid and adrenal problems, chronic fatigue, and memory impairment. It's tough to stick with a lifestyle change—or remember to do so—if poor indoor air quality drains your energy.

When the U.S. Environmental Protection Agency (EPA) conducted a survey of six hundred homes in six cities, researchers discovered that peak concentrations of twenty toxic compounds were hundreds of times higher inside homes than outside. "If we measured outdoors what we are measuring indoors," said EPA spokesperson Lance Wallace, "there would be a tremendous cry to clean up outdoor air."[14] The EPA ranks indoor air pollution as one of the five most urgent environmental problems facing this country.

My friend Dr. Joe Mercola points out that many homes have airborne pollutant levels twenty-five to one hundred times higher than the air outside the home. Since we spend so much time living inside confined spaces these days, a pollutant released indoors is a thousand times more likely to reach your lungs than a pollutant released outdoors.[15]

The remedy to poor air quality inside your home is to open your doors and windows several times a day to allow fresh air to flow into your home, no matter how cold or warm the temperature is outside. Even in Florida's sticky summer heat, Nicki and I periodically air out the house, and we have slept with a window cracked open in the master bedroom. We've also installed four air purifiers inside our home, which clean room air through electrical charges, capturing airborne particles, microbes, and molds.

Air purifiers are a wonderful technology that's becoming more affordable each year, but don't purchase ones that use ozone as their primary source of purification since overexposure to ozone can bring on asthma symptoms and even scar your lungs, according to Dr. Joe Mercola. You should also avoid ionic air purifiers, which don't remove much dust or come close to the performance of other air purifiers tested.

You also can take other steps around the house to improve your air quality. Change your air-conditioning and heater filters often. If possible, purchase highly efficient filters that trap micron-size particles. It's also imperative to wash your bed linens often—and your pillows. Dust mites by the hundreds of thousands and even millions camp out in sheets and pillowcases, according to the Mayo Clinic.[16] These microscopic creatures inhabit even the cleanest homes, and their residue—droppings and decaying carcasses—mixes with dust and becomes airborne. "If you aren't allergic to dust mite residue, it's not harmful," said the Mayo Clinic article. "But if you are, it can make you sneeze and wheeze year-round. Dust mites are one of the most common causes of perennial asthma and allergy symptoms."

Dust mites, which prefer warm environments, thrive just about anywhere inside the house: couches, carpets, stuffed toys, and bed covers. Their favorite abode are your sheets, where every evening is the grand opening of a warm, cozy, all-you-can-eat buffet of dead skin cells—yours.

While it's impossible to rid our homes of dust mites completely, you can take measures to diminish their numbers. Dusting and vacuuming once a week and doing a thorough job on the carpets, sofas, curtains, and blinds is an excellent start. Cut out the clutter by throwing out old newspapers and magazines and minimizing the knickknacks and tabletop ornaments gathering dust in your home. Wash sheets, pillowcases, and blankets weekly, and reduce the humidity with air conditioners and dehumidifiers to 50 percent or below, since dust mites shrivel up and die when they can't absorb moisture in the air. Finally, don't sleep in the same room as your dog or cat.

*Are You a Messie?*
*by Nicki Rubin*

Sandra Felton, who lives in south Florida, never threw out expired sales flyers that came with her junk mail. Why? Because when the next sale flyer arrived, she could tell if it would be better sale.

At least, that was her thinking. Meanwhile, she could never dig up those sales flyers from underneath the mounds of stacked papers, magazines, and newspapers lying around her house. Nor could she find a simple Band-Aid when one of the kids scraped a knee. Sandra was, in her own words, a "messie."

Part of reducing toxins in your environment is keeping a clean house, which rids living areas of microscopic dust mites and other critters. But messies and pack rats who can't bear to throw away old newspapers, magazines, and other "stuff" create an atmosphere where it's practically impossible to tidy up, vacuum carpets, or mop floors to any level of cleanliness.

Whether you're a messie or just living with one, you can turn things around. In Sandra's situation, she began by getting three boxes and labeling them "Throw Away," "Give Away," and "Store Elsewhere." Then she started cleaning up near the front door before gravitating to the first piece of furniture with a drawer.

She threw all the junk that had accumulated in the first drawer into the Throw Away box. She was serious about this. Sandra didn't keep the pen that worked half the time and the year-old calendar, even though it had nice pictures on it. Her freedom from clutter was more important than the freedom to hang on to an outdated calendar.

She didn't worry about cleaning walls, drapes, upholstery, and furniture during her first pass through the house. Basically, she organized one room in the house before going on to the next. When she had done enough for one day—about an hour or two—she stopped, put the boxes away, and picked up where she left off the following day.

Sandra did what she calls the "Mount Vernon" method of cleaning. At

George Washington's home, housekeepers arrive each morning and start at the front door, cleaning one room at a time. In other words, they finish one room before going on to the next. You should clean and organize one room at a time instead of straightening up part of the living room before tackling the stack of mail, papers, and bills atop the kitchen counter space. Cleaning and picking up around the house via the Mount Vernon method gives you a feeling of accomplishment and rids your home environment of unwanted toxins.[17]

Although indoor houseplants absorb their share of toxic compounds and pollutants and should be part of your home environment, don't go overboard with houseplants since they increase indoor humidity, which could lead to more dust mites. Still, I'm a fan of houseplants, especially after hearing about a National Aeronautics and Space Administration (NASA) study showing that indoor plants such as the English ivy, Chinese evergreen, and weeping fig can remove up to 87 percent of the toxins contained in indoor air.[18] Healthy, mature indoor plants not only clean up your indoor environment, but they add a lovely green accent to home furnishings.

In some parts of the country, a radon test is part of a home inspection before someone buys a home. Radon is a colorless, odorless gas that can be carcinogenic, and when radon levels are higher than U.S. government standards, the sellers are usually asked to pay for additional venting into the home—further proof that fresh air is a welcome antidote to toxins in the air we breathe.

You may not have paid much attention to the household cleaners beneath your kitchen sink or stored in bathroom cabinets. These cleaning products usually contain potentially harmful chemicals and solvents that expose people to VOCs (volatile organic compounds), which can cause eye, nose, and throat irritation. Furniture polish, air fresheners, adhesives, and household cleaners are filled with VOCs as well as semivolatile organic chemicals. Synthetic room fresheners and fragranced cleaning products are among the worst offenders, making indoor air unhealthy and provoking skin, eye, and respiratory reactions.

Since stay-at-home moms and preschool children spend 90 percent of their time indoors, according to the American Lung Association, you can see why this should be a concern. In homes where aerosol sprays and air fresheners were used frequently, mothers suffered 25 percent more headaches and 19 percent more depression, and infants under six months of age had 30 percent more ear infections and 22 percent higher incidence of diarrhea, according to a study done at Bristol University in England.[19]

I look to the *Safe Shopper's Bible*, coauthored by my good friend David Steinman, for recommendations regarding indoor air quality. First of all, you can quit buying air fresheners, deodorizers, and odor removers. Besides purchasing more indoor houseplants, you should bring home flower sachets and place them in strategic areas around the house. Health food stores also sell fragrance jars and dried botanicals.

**Nicki:** I can remember plugging those fragrance units into an outlet and thinking they made my apartment smell nice, but that's because I didn't know much about toxins inside a home environment. I discovered that scented candles were excellent substitutes for fragrance plug-ins, as well as beeswax candles, which are infused with essential oils and one of the healthiest type of candles you can bring into the home.

Fortunately, neither of us is chemically sensitive, but needlessly exposing ourselves to toxins didn't make sense. I found out that vinegar and water was good for cleaning kitchen countertops, windows, and fixtures. Jordan suggested that I try all-purpose cleaners from a company named Seventh Generation, and I immediately loved their household cleaning products and laundry detergent. Seventh Generation is an "alternative" brand that uses corn-, palm kernel–, or coconut-based oils, as well as replenishable and renewable resources instead of petrochemicals in formulating their products. Bi-O-Kleen, Orange TKO, and Aubrey Organics are also worth checking out. I recommend mops, wipes, and dusters from PerfectClean. These are available online at www.SixWise.com. PerfectClean mops and wipes come in an "ultramicrofiber" construction, which means you clean with just water—no chemical cleaners required.

These days, I do little things like wash my hand towels every couple of days and vacuum my carpet and tile floors with a vacuum cleaner that has a high-efficiency particulate air (HEPA) filter because contaminants often cling to household dust. These filters remove 99 percent of particles with a diameter greater than 0.3 microns.

**Jordan:** According to Philip Dickey of the Washington Toxics Coalition, the most hazardous and dangerous cleaning products are drain cleaners, oven cleaners, acidic toilet bowl cleaners, and anything containing chlorine or ammonia—which should never be combined, by the way.[20]

*The Green Guide* magazine did an excellent job of describing how to make your home naturally clean instead of a repository of chemical toxins. Here's a comprehensive list:

- **All-purpose cleaners and dish and laundry detergents.**

  Problem: These petroleum-based products contain phthalates, which are chemicals that have been linked to cancer in lab tests.

  Solution: Check out less toxic products from Ecover, Seventh Generation, Aubrey Organics, and Vermont Soapworks.
- **Antibacterial soaps and cleansers, bleach, stain removers, disinfectants, glass cleaners, and bathroom scouring powders.**

  Problem: Chlorine bleach, a common disinfectant, burns eyes and skin upon contact and is another suspected carcinogen. Many scouring powders and cleaning solutions contain bleach.

  Solution: White vinegar helps kill bacteria, mold, and viruses. A paste made from baking soda and water works effectively when scrubbing sinks, tubs, and countertops. Seventh Generation's sanitizers are also recommended.
- **Drain, oven, and toilet-bowl cleaners.**

  Problem: Horribly corrosive to the environment and can burn skin and eyes on contact.

Solution: For drains, have a plumber use a snake or try Earth Friendly or Naturally Yours drain cleaners. Ovens can be coated with a water and baking soda paste and allowed to stand overnight before being scrubbed off—with gloves on. Toilets clean up nicely with nonchlorine scouring powders like Ecover Toilet Cleaner.

- **Furniture and metal polishes.**

  Problem: They contain nerve-damaging petroleum distillates.

  Solution: Mix one teaspoon of olive oil and a half cup of white vinegar, or look for solvent-free products made from mineral or plant oils.

- **Room fresheners and other preformed products.**

  Problem: Fragrances can provoke allergic and asthmatic reactions.

  Solution: Open windows and let some fresh air in! Sachets of dried flowers or herbs provide gentle scents. Look for products scented with essential plant oils such as lemon, verbena, or lavender.[21]

Finally, there's one more household item that's a potential health hazard, and it's a nonstick frying pan. Pots and pans coated with Teflon or Teflon-like surfaces are immensely popular: 95 million nonstick pots and pans were purchased in 2004, according to the Cookware Manufacturers Association.[22]

While nonstick cookware has certainly made cleanup chores easier, scientific studies—as well as lawsuits—are suggesting that nonstick pots and pans give off potentially harmful fumes at medium to high temperatures.[23] In addition, a chemical crucial to the manufacture of nonstick surfaces—but not found in the finished pots and pans—is prevalent in the environment and in most Americans' blood.[24]

The scientific research regarding the dangers of nonstick cookware has prompted eight U.S. companies, including industry leader DuPont, to virtually eliminate a harmful chemical used to make Teflon from all consumer products by 2015. That chemical is called *perflorooctanoic acid*, or PFOA, and it has been linked to cancer and birth defects in animals and is in the blood of 95 percent of Americans, including pregnant women.[25]

Like the microwave, we've banished Teflon pots and pans from our home and recommend that you do the same. Stainless-steel and ceramic-coated metal cookware, as well as stoneware, are much safer for you. If you do cook with Teflon cookware, be sure to use coconut oil, which is more stable than vegetable oil, and be extra careful not to heat your food at high temperatures, since this appears to release more toxic particles into the air.

*Let There Be Light*
*by Jordan Rubin*

Back in the postwar 1940s, a photography buff named John Ott built a large greenhouse and hung cameras above the plants, recording the opening of the flowers by taking pictures seconds or minutes apart. When the images were put together as a sequence and played back on film, it gave the illusion of a flower opening up in seconds rather than hours. Ott was credited with inventing time-lapse photography.

A fellow named Walt Disney heard about Ott's invention and asked him to work on several Disney nature films, including *The Secrets of Life* and *Nature's Half-Acre*. While working with various kinds of lights for his flowers, Ott discovered that full-spectrum light—the same kind of light that streams from the sun—greatly enhanced plant growth. His plants did not grow as well under fluorescent lights, which is popular in offices and factories. Fluorescent light, he learned, emits light different from sunlight and is not as healthy as ultraviolet rays of sunlight, which provide a significant source of vitamin D.

John Ott became a proponent of full-spectrum light and devoted his remaining years to studying the healthy effects of sunlight and full-spectrum light. He recommended changing fluorescent or incandescent lighting to full-spectrum lighting, which, like sunlight, also produces ultraviolet rays.

Since we spend most of our time indoors and don't get the sunlight we should, I could see the benefits of switching over to full-spectrum lighting, which we did in the home we built last year. According to a *Wall Street Journal* report, a study by Pacific Gas and Electric found that sales increased an average of 40 percent in stores with skylights, and students in three states performed 10 to 20 percent better on tests under full-spectrum lighting conditions.[26] Full-spectrum lighting is more yellowish, just like the sun, and it makes reading easier with less eye strain.

## Water We Thinking?

**Jordan:** When snowbirds and tourists flock to Florida, they see numerous lakes and ponds dotting the landscape and experience the torrential thunderstorms in the summer—as well as Category 4 hurricanes that slam into the coastal areas, dumping ten to twenty inches of rain in twenty-four hours. Under those circumstances, most out-of-staters believe that Florida has an overabundance of fresh water for human consumption.

The reality is that Floridians face the same water shortages found in other regions of the country, despite the fact that our state receives 54 inches of rainfall per year on average. The trouble is that Floridians use more water per capita than residents of any other state except for California.[27]

Our water-management districts, in the interest of public safety, must treat our freshwater before releasing it into the municipal domestic-water pipeline. The first step involves adding chlorine or the chlorine alternative, *chloramine*, which is required by federal law, to kill disease-causing bacteria.

Water treatment is a complex process. Here's what happens to water before it reaches our taps:

- coagulation of contaminants using ferric sulfate and sulfuric acid to reduce naturally occurring organic matter
- flocculation (making small particles stick together into larger lumps) with polymer additives to reduce naturally occurring organics
- sedimentation to settle the flocculated particulates
- stabilization

- ozonation of the clear settled water (ozone is a strong oxidant that destroys harmful bacteria and viruses such as *Giardia* and *Crypto sporidium* as well as taste- and odor-causing compounds)
- addition of lime to the water to stabilize the pH of the treated water
- fluoridation (adding fluoride), which supposedly provides dental health benefits to water drinkers (though this has been the subject of much debate within the natural health community)
- disinfection by filtering through mixed-bed filters containing sand and activated carbon coal to remove remaining particles
- filtration, then addition of a chlorine-and-ammonia combination that produces a disinfectant called *monocloramine*, to "finish" the water and prepare it for storage
- addition of sodium hydroxide to produce the final desired drinking-water pH before storage in large cement underground tanks called "clear wells"[28]

Excuse me while I reach for a sip of Trinity Springs water, a bottled water that comes from a natural spring lacking the chemistry of municipal tap water. Let's put it this way: I try to never, ever drink tap water. This is why I installed a whole-house water filtration in our garage. When municipal water—already treated with enough chemical compounds to open a pool-supply store—reaches our property, our filtration system removes the chlorine and other impurities before the water enters our household pipes. My family can confidently drink filtered water from every tap in our home, and our foods can be washed and cooked in filtered water as well.

An in-home water filtering system involves an investment of several thousand dollars, depending on the size of your home. You don't have to spend a lot of money, however, to dramatically improve the quality of water inside the home. A countertop water pitcher with a built-in carbon-based filter costs between $20 and $40, and installing water filters at your kitchen sink and in the bathrooms is reasonable as well.

If you can only install one water filter inside your home, put it on your showerhead. Did you know that standing beneath a steaming spray of shower water is the chlorine equivalent to drinking six to eight glasses of chlorinated water? That's how much chlorine the skin, whose pores are opened up by the beading of hot water, soaks up, along with the amount of chlorine, which is a gas, is inhaled.

Chlorine is a powerful chemical, hard on your skin as well as your hair because of the way chlorine bonds with hair and breaks down protein, making hair dry and brittle and causing itchy skin and flaky scalp. Showering in chlorinated water exposes your skin to a relatively large volume of a diluted chlorine solution, which reacts to the oils in the skin to form chlorinated compounds that may be absorbed by the body. Regular exposure to chlorinated water promotes the aging process of the skin, not unlike extended exposure to sunlight.

Shower filters range from inexpensive carbon-block sieves similar to countertop water pitchers to more sophisticated kinetic degradation fluxion (KDF) units, which contain a special high-purity alloy that removes chlorine, heavy metals, and bacteria from the water. Once installed, these shower filters remove the toxic burden for a year until the filter needs to be changed.

If you prefer to soak in a hot bath, bath filter balls float in the tub and reportedly remove 90 percent of the chlorine in the water. (For more information on water filtration products, visit www.BiblicalHealthInsitute.com and click on the GPRx Resource Guide.)

## Feminine Hygiene and Beauty

Let's switch gears and talk about going organic when it comes to using unbleached toilet paper and uh . . . feminine hygiene products. Back in the 1980s, toxic shock syndrome (TSS) killed dozens of women. The syndrome was linked to overabsorbent tampons that created a breeding ground for the bacteria called *Staphlococcus aureas.* Lately, according to a University of Minnesota study, toxic shock syndrome is making a comeback, although not a serious charge.[29] Women are advised to use the lowest-absorbency tampon possible and change tampons every four hours. Medical attention should be sought if you experience high fever, chills, vomiting, diarrhea, or a rash. During toxic shock, blood pressure drops to dangerously low levels.

I think women should consider using organic/unbleached toilet paper and tampons. Many conventional feminine care products are made with absorbent fibers that have been bleached with chlorine, which, as I just described, is a toxin you want to avoid. Toilet paper and tampons made from 100 percent certified organic cotton and whitened without chlorine are safer for sensitive skin and free of irritating dyes or fragrances. Also, using organic cotton products keeps the amount of dangerous chlorinated toxins and pesticide residues out of your body. An excellent producer of organic toilet paper and tampons is a company called Seventh Generation (www.seventhgeneration.com).

**Nicki:** I've pretty much switched over to organic when it comes to facial cleansers, toners, body lotions, and moisturizers too. Shampoo, hairspray, and makeup have been a different story for me, however. Even though I've tried to find products I like at the health food store, it's been difficult to locate something better than my favorite shampoo that I've used for years. Hairspray from the health food store also tends to be very sticky, and I don't go for the crunchy hair look. I prefer hairspray that I can barely feel after I apply it because I like the feel of real hair on my head. Although I use the least amount of hairspray as possible, Jordan doesn't want to be in the bathroom or master bedroom when I spray, so I have to warn him before I use it.

As for cosmetics, I use Lancôme for my mascara, lipstick, and lip liner. Again, I haven't been able to find organic makeup or hairspray that I like, but as with hairspray, I will continue searching, as I know I should be avoiding the toxins that these products contain. One of the advantages of staying home with Joshua is that I don't have to wear makeup most of the time, but when I go out, I wear it.

**Jordan:** *The Safe Shopper's Bible* points out that cosmetics have been used for thousands of years—even before written history—for beauty, power, and heightened sexuality.[30] While privileged women in the ancient empires of Egypt, Greece, and Rome used a variety of minerals and natural compounds to darken their eyelashes and eyebrows and color their lips, they also relied on more toxic substances to give them the right look for the vernal equinox festival or race day at the Colosseum. Egyptian women used lead sulfate for painting the upper eyelids black. In Athens, women colored their lips and painted their eyebrows with charcoal pencils, and in Caesar's time, upscale Roman women used toxic mercury compounds for tinting and white lead to whiten their skin.[31]

Not much has changed in two thousand years.

When I speak at women's conferences, I tell women straight out that I will not put anything on my skin that I would not eat. That's because the skin is superabsorbent, and a good way to prove that is to rub some crushed garlic on the soles of your feet. Take it from someone who danced at a friend's wedding smelling like a vat of fresh garlic: after rubbing your feet with garlic cloves, you'll be running to the bathroom within twenty minutes to brush your teeth because you'll smell garlic on your breath. Similarly, when you rub a tube of lipstick across your lips, you're introducing potentially damaging agents to your bloodstream.

Toxic chemicals are plentiful in our everyday cosmetics and toiletries. Products such as lipstick, lip gloss, lip conditioner, hair coloring, hairspray, shampoo, and soap routinely contain chemical solvents and phthalates, though you could never tell from reading the labels. That's because the long list of ingredients contain multisyllabic words that defy pronunciation, let alone comprehension, by the average consumer. Nowhere on the label will you find an explanation of how these ingredients work, leaving health-conscious women in the dark.

Let me shine some light on the situation. Phthalates are chemicals with many industrial uses, including being used to preserve cosmetics and fragrances. Emerging scientific evidence is raising serious concerns, as certain phthalates have been shown to cause a wide range of adverse effects in laboratory animals, including reproductive and developmental harm, organ damage, endocrine disruption, and cancer. From the industry side, the phthalate producers counter that human exposure levels are far below minimum safety levels set by U.S. regulatory agencies.

Your goal should be to minimize your exposure to potentially harmful toxins in our environment whenever and wherever you can. Natural cosmetics without phthalates can be found in progressive grocery and natural food stores, but they are becoming much more widely available in drugstores, supermarkets, and beauty stores in malls.

Even using underarm antiperspirant could heighten the risk of breast cancer. Antiperspirants contain chemicals, such as aluminum salts, that mimic the body's natural hormone estrogen, which are known to affect breast cancer risk.[32] Researchers are studying antiperspirants because they are used so closely to the breast and are often used by women directly after shaving, which might allow for easier absorption. Consider using antiperspirants (which stop perspiration) or deodorants (which mask odor) found in natural food stores. For information on our favorite personal care products, visit www.BiblicalHealthInstitute.com and click on the GPRx Resource Guide.

**Nicki:** Like I said, it's been a challenge to find organic substitutes for everyday cosmetics and toiletries, but I expect organic skin cosmetics to improve as the market for them grows bigger. I'm hoping that Jordan and his research team will develop more effective and usable products, which I believe are in the works as we speak. I agree with Jordan that it's a worthwhile goal to minimize your exposure to potentially harmful toxins whenever you can.

**Jordan:** In the future, organic soaps, shampoos, and skin creams should become easier to find since the U.S. Agricultural Department's National Organic Program declared in 2005 that cosmetics can be labeled with the "USDA Organic" green seal—as long as 95 percent of the ingredients are organic. Without the USDA requirements, there would be anarchy in product labeling, said Craig Minowa, an environmental scientist for the Organic Consumers Association. "Now consumers can look for the USDA seal and know the product has met tough standards."[33]

## Breast Health

Every time I thumb through a glossy magazine from the Miami area, it seems as though every other page contains an advertisement for breast augmentation surgery. Along South Beach, deep tans and fit bodies are worshipped, and many less-endowed women—for a variety of reasons—feel compelled to enhance what God gave them through breast implants. Botox injections and liposuction are popular as well.

Talk about introducing environmental toxins into your body. The Food and Drug Administration banned silicone-gel implants in 1992 (except for mastectomy patients) following a wave of lawsuits, including a famous one involving Dow Chemical, the maker of a silicone breast implant. The company lost a multimillion-dollar judgment when a woman claimed her implants caused an autoimmune disorder; Dow Chemical later filed for bankruptcy protection in 1995 to shield itself from tens of thousands of other lawsuits related to its breast implants.[34]

Saline breast implants, which have a silicone rubber shell and are inflated to desired size with sterile saline, were the only FDA-approved breast implants following the ban on silicone breast implants. (That changed in 2005 when the FDA approved silicone gel-filled implants produced by Mentor and Inamed.) For a variety of reasons, mainly cultural, breast augmentation surgery has become very popular in the last ten years. More than 264,000 breast-implant surgeries were performed for purely cosmetic reasons in 2004, according to the American Society of Plastic Surgeons,[35] twice the number done in 1998.

Suddenly, everyone from Hollywood starlets to soccer moms is scheduling appointments with plastic surgeons. The rumor in south Florida's snazzier zip codes is that high-school girls are asking for breast-enhancement surgery as a graduation present, which partially explains why the number of teenage girls nationwide having breast augmentation has quadrupled since the late 1990s.[36] Young women are no doubt influenced by TV reality shows like *The Swan* and E! Channel's *Doctor 90210*, which has a Beverly Hills plastic surgeon saying to the camera, "If you're not a double-D, come see me."

My feelings on breast implants are the same as on botox injections: be very wary about introducing silicone, saline, or tattoo ink, for that matter, into your body. Nicki and I understand that there are women reading this book who have undergone breast implant surgery—or gotten a tattoo or two—and we are not attempting to pass judgment on such private decisions. What we're saying is that there is a lot of smoke around the dangers of breast implants, botox injections, liposuction, and tattoos. And the jury is still out on the long-term complications associated with breast implant surgery, such as implant leakage, deflation, and repeat operations. Tattoos and other forms of "body art" are often done in parlors that are unregulated, unsanitary, and undependable. Those on the sharp end of a tattoo needle risk infection for everything from hepatitis B to HIV.

The moral of the story is to be careful and become informed. Read everything you can on the subject before making a decision to proceed.

**Nicki:** Breast implants are all over TV, and they make it sound like it's nothing more than having your nails done, but it's far more than that, of course. Now I'd like to turn the discussion to something that Jordan talked about in the Introduction, which is breast cancer. We've all heard the tragic stories of a young mother losing a brave battle to the deadly disease, leaving behind a grieving husband and children who can't understand why Mommy had to die. Perhaps you have a family member or a close friend who passed away or had a battle with breast cancer.

**Jordan:** I have no doubt that environmental factors have contributed to the high numbers of women who develop breast cancer. Over 211,000 new cases of invasive breast cancer were diagnosed in 2005.[37] Yes, genetics and family history do play a role (between 5 and 10 percent of all cancers are clearly hereditary), but the choices in the food we eat, the amount of time we exercise, the hygiene we practice, the stress we undergo, and the otherwise imbalanced lives we lead account for about 65 percent of cancer deaths in the United States, according to the Harvard University School of Public Health.[38]

**Nicki:** Breast health is important to a woman's self-esteem and her sexual self-image. While God designed the female breast to provide optimal nourishment for babies, the bosom symbolizes many things to a woman: femininity, beauty, attractiveness, nurturance, motherhood, and yes, sexuality.

The importance of breast health is underscored in a marital relationship. The loss or alteration of a breast through a mastectomy or lumpectomy—the common surgical techniques to fight breast cancer—affects every husband and wife and their sexual relationship. While doctors have not yet discovered the cause of breast cancer, they do know that cancer cells form a lump or mass in the breast, prompting a benign or malignant tumor to grow. Benign tumors are not cancerous or life threatening, but a malignant tumor can travel fairly rapidly to others parts of the body. A heightened awareness of breast changes or skin changes may result in early detection of tumors. When breast cancer has grown to the point where physical symptoms exist, you might detect a lump, thickening, swelling, distortion, or tenderness.

*A Primer on Breast Self-Exams*
*by Pancheta Wilson, MD*

A breast self-examination should be done monthly, about five days after menstruation, when the breasts are less swollen and tender. (After menopause, a breast self-exam should be done at the same time each month, using your calendar to remind you.) Changes in the breast are found more easily when examining your breast in the shower with a soapy hand. You can also stand before a mirror and hold one arm high while the other hand searches the breast for a lump or hard knot. Other things to look for are changes in the nipple, such as an indrawn or dimpled look. Any difference in the pigmentation or texture of the breast, such as a reddish, pitted surface, like the skin of an orange, is another potential breast cancer symptom.

A highly regarded breast self-exam developed by University of Florida researchers is called the MammaCare method. The woman should lie down on a bed, pull her knees up slightly, and place her left hand palm up on her fore head. Then she uses her right hand to examine her left breast, first by lying on her right side, and then by lying flat on her back. The side-lying position allows a woman, especially one with large breasts, to perform an effective examination. Once lying on her back, the woman should feel for any lumps from her bra line to the middle of her breastbone.

There's no doubt that breast cancer is a modern-day plague and elicits feelings of dread and concern. Fortunately, advancements in modern medicine can protect us from the ravages of cancer, and exciting changes in surgical techniques, radiation, and chemotherapy treatments have vastly improved the chances of survivability. The five-year survival rate for most breast cancers is 85 percent, a result tagged to regular cancer screening. But though improving survival rates are comforting, cancer remains a ruthless killer. For those who survive and experience remission (and lose all their hair as well as their sense of taste), the slash-and-burn cure can be worse than the disease. Modern cancer treatment revolves around two extremely unpleasant options: radiation and chemotherapy. That's why I feel deeply for anyone diagnosed with this dreadful disease.

I have difficultly imagining the private horror of sitting across the desk from an oncologist, nervously working a Kleenex in your hands, anxiously awaiting the verdict. What do people think after the doctor glances at the medical reports, stiffly clears her throat, and wearily announces, "I regret to inform you that you have cancer"? I hope to spare you—and myself—from ever hearing those life-changing words, and I believe the seven keys of the Great Physician's prescription offer you a straight path to minimize the considerable risk that you may one day develop cancer in your body.

If you have heard those same words directed to you, then please know that you have my complete sympathy. The phrase "I know what you're going through" is not applicable here because I *don't* know what it's like to be told I have cancer. But this is one disease where an ounce of prevention is worth far more than a ton of cure, to quote an old proverb.

I believe with all my heart that by following these Seven Keys, your battle against breast cancer will have a much greater chance to end in victory. For more information on a battle plan geared specifically to cancer, read *The Great Physician's Rx for Cancer.*

*What Women Are Saying*
*by Denise Vance*

About five years ago, I began experiencing very severe sinus headaches in my eyebrow and upper cheekbone area, as well an overall feeling of lethargy; I couldn't read because the headaches were so bad. My symptoms were so strong and painful that I had difficulty expressing how awful I felt to my friends.

I sought help from my doctors, who examined me for allergies. They told me I was allergic to pollen, dust mites, cats, dogs, and every kind of grass but juniper. They prescribed allergy medications, which, at the beginning, helped me make it through the day. By 8 p.m., however, I was so bone tired that I had to go straight to bed. I usually slept straight through the night because of my exhaustion.

Something was really wrong with me, so when the allergy medications lost their effectiveness, my doctors suggested adding allergy shots to my regimen. Once or twice a week, I would go to the doctor's office for another allergy shot.

My poor husband, Dale. He'd come home from work and peek into the master bedroom, where I would be sound asleep at 8:05 p.m. You could say that my allergies were affecting my marriage in more ways than one.

I prayed a lot during this time, when illness consumed my life. I thought, *God, what is this? Can you show me how this can be resolved? I can't go on like this, and neither can my family.*

Then I heard about Jordan Rubin and the Great Physician's Rx. The advanced hygiene program caught my attention right away because within a couple of days, I noticed a big change in my allergies. The congestion in my head cleared up. I could take a full, complete breath without developing a splitting headache. I noticed that practicing advanced hygiene before bed was great, and it helped me breathe better at night.

I was turning a corner.

I was able to get off allergy medications completely—after I made the switch to eating God's way. That part was fun for me because I like to cook, but I had a "lightbulb" moment when I realized that when we prayed for God to bless our food, then our food better be wholesome and healthy, or why ask Him to bless it? I couldn't pray, *Lord, bless this icky food that we are about to put into our mouths and use it to nourish our bodies.*

Now when Dale or I say grace before meals, we can honestly thank God with a grateful heart that He has provided something far healthier than what we used to eat, and that's something worth thanking Him for.

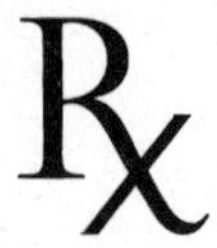

## THE GREAT PHYSICIAN'S Rx FOR WOMEN'S HEALTH: REDUCE TOXINS IN YOUR ENVIRONMENT

- *If you're on hormone replacement therapy (HRT) medications, talk to your health-care provider about using a more natural substitute.*
- *Consume organically produced food as much as possible, and stay away from processed foods, which are often made from genetically modified crops.*
- *Stay away from low-calorie and no-calorie artificial sweeteners.*
- *Improve indoor air quality by opening windows, changing air filters regularly, setting out houseplants, and buying an air filtration system.*

- *Don't cook with microwave ovens.*
- *Switch from fluorescent to full-spectrum lighting.*
- *Consider purchasing a water filtration system for your home so you and your family can drink and shower in purified water.*
- *Use natural skin care, body, hair, cosmetic, and feminine hygiene products.*
- *Don't cook with nonstick cookware made of aluminum, which can give off potentially harmful toxins when heated.*
- *Use natural cleaning products for your home, washer, and dishwasher.*
- *Practice good breast health by performing regular self-exams.*

## THE GREAT PHYSICIAN'S RX FOR WEEK #5

Remember to visit www.BiblicalHealthInstitute.com and click on the GPRx Resource Guide to learn more about the foods, supplements, advanced hygiene products, exercise and body therapy resources, and products to help reduce toxins in your environment, that we recommend in the Great Physician's Rx 7 Weeks of Wellness plan.

### DAY 29

*You will notice that some items in the meal plans that follow are italicized. You can find the recipes for these—and over other 250 delicious and healthy recipes—at www.BiblicalHealthInstitute.com.*

### *Upon Waking*

*Advanced hygiene:* Practice advanced hygiene. See page 277 for guidance.

*Reduce toxins:* Open windows for one hour today. Make a plan to change air-conditioning or heating filters more regularly.

*Supplements:* Take one serving of a fiber/green superfood combination containing ground flaxseed, mixed in 12 to 16 ounces of water or raw vegetable juice.

*Body therapy:* Take a hot-and-cold shower. After normal shower, alternate sixty seconds of water as hot as you can stand it, followed by sixty seconds of water as cold as you can stand it. Repeat cycle four times for a total of eight minutes, finishing with cold.

*Exercise:* Perform functional fitness exercises for fifteen minutes, or spend fifteen minutes on the rebounder. Finish with ten minutes of deep-breathing exercises. During exercise, drink 8 ounces of water.

### *Breakfast*

During breakfast, drink 8 ounces of water.

two eggs (omega-3 or organic, and prepared as desired)

one piece of fruit

one piece of whole-grain sprouted or sourdough toast with butter

hot tea with honey

*Supplements:* Take two whole food multivitamin caplets, one capsule of omega-3 cod-liver oil, and two caplets of a whole food calcium/magnesium blend.

### *Between Breakfast and Lunch*

Drink 12 ounces of water.

### *Lunch*

During lunch, drink 8 ounces of water.

green salad with two hard-boiled omega-3 eggs, carrots, red onions, cucumbers, and yellow peppers

healthy salad dressing with one tablespoon of extra-virgin olive oil or high-lignan flaxseed oil

one piece of fruit

*Supplements:* Take two whole food multivitamin caplets, one capsule of omega-3 cod-liver oil, and two caplets of a whole food calcium/magnesium blend.

***Between Lunch and Dinner***

Drink 12 ounces of water.

***Dinner***

During dinner, drink 8 ounces of water.

fish of choice

baked white potato (organic)

green salad with red or yellow peppers, red onions, green or red cabbage, celery, cucumbers, and carrots

healthy salad dressing with olive oil and/or high-lignan flaxseed oil

*Supplements:* Take two whole food multivitamin caplets, one capsule of omega-3 cod-liver oil, and two caplets of a whole food calcium/magnesium blend.

***Snack/Dessert***

apple cinnamon whole food bar (with beta-glucans from soluble oat fiber)

whole-milk yogurt, fruit, and honey

***Before Bed***

*Exercise:* Go for a walk outdoors or participate in a favorite sport or recreational activity. During exercise, drink 8 ounces of water.

*Supplements:* Take one serving of a fiber/green superfood combination containing ground flaxseed, mixed in 12 to 16 ounces of water or raw vegetable juice.

*Advanced hygiene:* Practice advanced hygiene.

*Body therapy:* Spend ten minutes listening to soothing music before you retire.

*Sleep:* Go to bed by 10:30 p.m.

## DAY 30

*You will notice that some items in the meal plans that follow are italicized. You can find the recipes for these—and over other 250 delicious and healthy recipes—at www.BiblicalHealthInstitute.com.*

### *Upon Waking*

*Advanced hygiene:* Practice advanced hygiene. See page 277 for guidance.

*Reduce toxins:* Open windows for one hour today. Purchase three houseplants and place them in your living room and dining area.

*Supplements:* Take one serving of a fiber/green superfood combination containing ground flaxseed, mixed in 12 to 16 ounces of water or raw vegetable juice.

*Body therapy:* Get twenty minutes of direct sunlight.

*Exercise:* Perform functional fitness exercises for fifteen minutes, or spend fifteen minutes on the rebounder. Finish with ten minutes of deep-breathing exercises. During exercise, drink 8 ounces of water.

### *Breakfast*

During breakfast, drink 8 ounces of water.

For a healthy smoothie, mix the following in a blender:

8 ounces plain whole milk, yogurt, or kefir

1 tablespoon honey

1/2 cup fresh or frozen fruit (bananas, peaches, berries, pineapple, etc.)

1 teaspoon high-lignan flaxseed oil

1 serving of protein powder (optional)

*Supplements:* Take two whole food multivitamin caplets, one capsule of omega-3 cod-liver oil, and two caplets of a whole food calcium/magnesium blend.

### *Between Breakfast and Lunch*

Drink 12 ounces of water.

***Lunch***

During lunch, drink 8 ounces of water.

low-mercury, high omega-3 tuna on sprouted or yeast-free whole-grain bread, with lettuce, tomato, and sprouts

one piece of fruit

*Supplements:* Take two whole food multivitamin caplets, one capsule of omega-3 cod-liver oil, and two caplets of a whole food calcium/magnesium blend.

***Between Lunch and Dinner***

Drink 12 ounces of water.

***Dinner***

During dinner, drink 8 ounces of water.

*Cilantro-Lime Halibut*

sautéed asparagus and mushrooms

couscous

*Supplements:* Take two whole food multivitamin caplets, one capsule of omega-3 cod-liver oil, and two caplets of a whole food calcium/magnesium blend.

***Snack/Dessert***

whole food meal replacement powder (with beta-glucans from soluble oat fiber) mixed in 12 ounces of water

one piece of fruit and 1 ounce of cheese

***Before Bed***

*Exercise:* Go for a walk outdoors or participate in a favorite sport or recreational activity. During exercise, drink 8 ounces of water.

*Supplements:* Take one serving of a fiber/green superfood combination containing ground flaxseed, mixed in 12 to 16 ounces of water or raw vegetable juice.

*Body therapy:* Take a warm bath, with eight drops of biblical essential oils added, for fifteen minutes.

*Advanced hygiene:* Practice advanced hygiene.

*Sleep:* Go to bed by 10:30 p.m.

## DAY 31

*You will notice that some items in the meal plans that follow are italicized. You can find the recipes for these—and over other 250 delicious and healthy recipes—at www.BiblicalHealthInstitute.com.*

### *Upon Waking*

*Advanced hygiene:* Practice advanced hygiene. See page 277 for guidance.

*Reduce toxins:* Open windows for one hour today. Purchase and install carbon-block shower filters for each shower in your home (if you're on city water).

*Supplements:* Take one serving of a fiber/green superfood combination containing ground flaxseed, mixed in 12 to 16 ounces of water or raw vegetable juice.

*Body therapy:* Take a hot-and-cold shower.

*Exercise:* Perform functional fitness exercises for fifteen minutes, or spend fifteen minutes on the rebounder. Finish with ten minutes of deep-breathing exercises. During exercise, drink 8 ounces of water.

### *Breakfast*

During breakfast, drink 8 ounces of water.

sprouted dry cereal with yogurt, goat's milk, or almond milk

banana

hot tea with honey

*Supplements:* Take two whole food multivitamin caplets, one capsule of omega-3 cod-liver oil, and two caplets of a whole food calcium/magnesium blend.

### *Between Breakfast and Lunch*

Drink 12 ounces of water.

*Lunch*

During lunch, drink 8 ounces of water.

green salad with 3 ounces of tuna (low-mercury, high omega-3) and carrots, red onions, cucumbers, and yellow peppers

healthy salad dressing with one tablespoon of extra-virgin olive oil or high-lignan flaxseed oil

one piece of fruit

*Supplements:* Take two whole food multivitamin caplets, one capsule of omega-3 cod-liver oil, and two caplets of a whole food calcium/magnesium blend.

*Between Lunch and Dinner*

Drink 12 ounces of water.

*Dinner*

During dinner, drink 8 ounces of water.

*Nicki's Meatloaf*

*Garlic Mashed Potatoes*

peas and carrots

*Supplements:* Take two whole food multivitamin caplets, one capsule of omega-3 cod-liver oil, and two caplets of a whole food calcium/magnesium blend.

*Snack/Dessert*

berry antioxidant whole food bar (with beta-glucans from soluble oat fiber)

apple and almond or sesame butter (tahini)

*Before Bed*

*Exercise:* Go for a walk outdoors or participate in a favorite sport or recreational activity. During exercise, drink 8 ounces of water.

*Supplements:* Take one serving of a fiber/green superfood combination containing ground flaxseed, mixed in 12 to 16 ounces of water or raw vegetable juice.

*Advanced hygiene:* Practice advanced hygiene.

*Body therapy:* Spend ten minutes listening to soothing music before you retire.

*Sleep:* Go to bed by 10:30 p.m.

## DAY 32

*You will notice that some items in the meal plans that follow are italicized. You can find the recipes for these—and over other 250 delicious and healthy recipes—at www.BiblicalHealthInstitute.com.*

### *Upon Waking*

*Advanced hygiene:* Practice advanced hygiene. See page 277 for guidance.

*Reduce toxins:* Open windows for one hour today. Use natural soap and natural skin and body care products (shower gel, body creams, etc.).

*Supplements:* Take one serving of a fiber/green superfood combination containing ground flaxseed, mixed in 12 to 16 ounces of water or raw vegetable juice.

*Body therapy:* Get twenty minutes of direct sunlight.

*Exercise:* Perform functional fitness exercises for fifteen minutes, or spend fifteen minutes on the rebounder. Finish with ten minutes of deep-breathing exercises. During exercise, drink 8 ounces of water.

### *Breakfast*

During breakfast, drink 8 ounces of water.

For a healthy smoothie, mix the following in a blender:

8 ounces plain whole milk, yogurt, or kefir

1 tablespoon honey

1/2 cup fresh or frozen fruit (bananas, peaches, berries, pineapple, etc.)

1 teaspoon high-lignan flaxseed oil

1 serving of protein powder (optional)

*Supplements:* Take two whole food multivitamin caplets, one capsule of omega-3 cod-liver oil, and two caplets of a whole food calcium/magnesium blend.

### *Between Breakfast and Lunch*

Drink 12 ounces of water.

*Lunch*

During lunch, drink 8 ounces of water.

turkey on sprouted or yeast-free whole-grain bread, with lettuce, tomato, and sprouts

one piece of fruit

*Supplements:* Take two whole food multivitamin caplets, one capsule of omega-3 cod-liver oil, and two caplets of a whole food calcium/magnesium blend.

*Between Lunch and Dinner*

Drink 12 ounces of water.

*Dinner*

During dinner, drink 8 ounces of water.

*Herb Stir-Fried Chicken and Mixed Veggies*

steamed broccoli

green salad with red or yellow peppers, red onions, green or red cabbage, celery, cucumbers, and carrots

healthy salad dressing with olive oil and/or high-lignan flaxseed oil

*Supplements:* Take two whole food multivitamin caplets, one capsule of omega-3 cod-liver oil, and two caplets of a whole food calcium/magnesium blend.

*Snack/Dessert*

whole food meal replacement powder (with beta-glucans from soluble oat fiber) mixed in 12 ounces of water

raw veggies and hummus, salsa, or guacamole

*Before Bed*

*Exercise:* Go for a walk outdoors or participate in a favorite sport or recreational activity. During exercise, drink 8 ounces of water.

*Supplements:* Take one serving of a fiber/green superfood combination containing ground flaxseed, mixed in 12 to 16 ounces of water or raw vegetable juice.

*Body therapy:* Take a warm bath, with eight drops of biblical essential oils added, for fifteen minutes.

*Advanced hygiene:* Practice advanced hygiene.

*Sleep:* Go to bed by 10:30 p.m.

## DAY 33 (PARTIAL-FAST DAY)

*You will notice that some items in the meal plans that follow are italicized. You can find the recipes for these—and over other 250 delicious and healthy recipes—at www.BiblicalHealthInstitute.com.*

***Upon Waking***

*Advanced hygiene:* Practice advanced hygiene. See page 277 for guidance.

*Reduce toxins:* Open windows for one hour today. Use natural soap and natural skin and body care products (shower gel, body creams, etc.).

*Supplements:* Take one serving of a fiber/green superfood combination containing ground flaxseed, mixed in 12 to 16 ounces of water or raw vegetable juice.

*Body therapy:* Take a hot-and-cold shower.

*Exercise:* Perform functional fitness exercises for fifteen minutes, or spend fifteen minutes on the rebounder. Finish with ten minutes of deep-breathing exercises. During exercise, drink 8 ounces of water.

***Breakfast***

none (partial-fast day)

Drink 12 ounces of water.

***Between Breakfast and Lunch***

Drink 12 ounces of water.

***Lunch***

none (partial-fast day)

Drink 12 ounces of water.

***Between Lunch and Dinner***

Drink 12 ounces of water.

***Dinner***

During dinner, drink 8 ounces of water.

*Chicken Soup*

wild salmon

fermented vegetables

green salad with red or yellow peppers, red onions, green or red cabbage, celery, cucumbers, and carrots

healthy salad dressing with olive oil and/or high-lignan flaxseed oil

*Supplements:* Take two whole food multivitamin caplets, one capsule of omega-3 cod-liver oil, and two caplets of a whole food calcium/magnesium blend.

***Snack/Dessert***

none (partial-fast day)

Drink twelve ounces of water

***Before Bed***

*Exercise:* Go for a walk outdoors or participate in a favorite sport or recreational activity. During exercise, drink 8 ounces of water.

*Supplements:* Take one serving of a fiber/green superfood combination containing ground flaxseed, mixed in 12 to 16 ounces of water or raw vegetable juice.

*Advanced hygiene:* Practice advanced hygiene. See page 277 for guidance.

*Body therapy:* Spend ten minutes listening to soothing music before you retire.

*Sleep:* Go to bed by 10:30 p.m.

## DAY 34 (DAY OF REST)

*You will notice that some items in the meal plans that follow are italicized. You can find the recipes for these—and over other 250 delicious and healthy recipes—at www.BiblicalHealthInstitute.com.*

***Upon Waking***

*Advanced hygiene:* Practice advanced hygiene. See page 277 for guidance.

*Reduce toxins:* Open windows for one hour today. Use natural soap, natural skin and body care products, and natural facial care products. Purchase and begin using natural toothpaste.

*Supplements:* Take one serving of a fiber/green superfood combination containing ground flaxseed, mixed in 12 to 16 ounces of water or raw vegetable juice.

*Exercise:* do no formal exercise since it's a day of rest.

*Body therapies:* do none since it's a rest day.

***Breakfast***

During breakfast, drink 8 ounces of water.

sprouted or raw dry cereal

4 ounces of whole-milk yogurt or goat's milk

raw honey

fresh fruit

hot tea with honey

Supplements: Take two whole food multivitamin caplets, one capsule of omega-3 cod-liver oil, and two caplets of a whole food calcium/magnesium blend.

***Between Breakfast and Lunch***

Drink 12 ounces of water.

***Lunch***

During lunch, drink 8 ounces of water.

green salad with 3 ounces of salmon, and carrots, red onions, cucumbers, and yellow peppers

healthy salad dressing with one tablespoon of extra-virgin olive oil or high-lignan flaxseed oil

one piece of fruit

Supplements: Take two whole food multivitamin caplets, one capsule of omega-3 cod-liver oil, and two caplets of a whole food calcium/magnesium blend.

***Between Lunch and Dinner***

Drink 12 ounces of water.

***Dinner***

During dinner, drink 8 ounces of water.

*Mushroom Soup*

chicken of choice

green salad with red or yellow peppers, red onions, green or red cabbage, celery, cucumbers, and carrots

healthy salad dressing with olive oil and/or high-lignan flaxseed oil

*Supplements:* Take two whole food multivitamin caplets, one capsule of omega-3 cod-liver oil, and two caplets of a whole food calcium/magnesium blend.

***Snack/Dessert***

green superfood whole food bar (with beta-glucans from soluble oat fiber)

soaked/sprouted dehydrated nuts and seeds

***Before Bed***

*Exercise:* do no formal exercise since it's a day of rest.

*Body therapies*: do none since it's a rest day.

*Supplements:* Take one serving of a fiber/green superfood combination containing ground flaxseed, mixed in 12 to 16 ounces of water or raw vegetable juice.

*Advanced hygiene:* Practice advanced hygiene.

*Sleep:* Go to bed by 10:30 p.m.

## DAY 35

*You will notice that some items in the meal plans that follow are italicized. You can find the recipes for these—and over other 250 delicious and healthy recipes—at www.BiblicalHealthInstitute.com.*

***Upon Waking***

*Advanced hygiene:* Practice advanced hygiene. See page 277 for guidance.

*Reduce toxins:* Open windows for one hour today. Use all-natural soap, skin and body care products, facial care products, and toothpaste. Purchase and begin using natural hair care products, such as shampoo, conditioner, gel, mousse, and hairspray.

*Supplements:* Take one serving of a fiber/green superfood combination containing ground flaxseed, mixed in 12 to 16 ounces of water or raw vegetable juice.

*Body therapy:* Get twenty minutes of direct sunlight.

*Exercise:* Perform functional fitness exercises for fifteen minutes, or spend fifteen minutes on the rebounder. Finish with ten minutes of deep-breathing exercises. During exercise, drink 8 ounces of water.

***Breakfast***

During breakfast, drink 8 ounces of water.

two-egg omelet with avocado, cheese, tomato, onion, and pepper

*Sautéed Veggies*

hot tea and honey

*Supplements:* Take two whole food multivitamin caplets, one capsule of omega-3 cod-liver oil, and two caplets of a whole food calcium/magnesium blend.

***Between Breakfast and Lunch***

Drink 12 ounces of water.

***Lunch***

During lunch, drink 8 ounces of water.

almond butter and honey or pure fruit jam on sprouted or yeast-free whole-grain bread

one piece of fruit

*Supplements:* Take two whole food multivitamin caplets, one capsule of omega-3 cod-liver oil, and two caplets of a whole food calcium/magnesium blend.

***Between Lunch and Dinner***

Drink 12 ounces of water.

***Dinner***

During dinner, drink 8 ounces of water.

ground bison patties with grilled onions and mushrooms

baked sweet potato with butter

green beans

*Supplements:* Take two whole food multivitamin caplets, one capsule of omega-3 cod-liver oil, and two caplets of a whole food calcium/magnesium blend.

***Snack/Dessert***

whole food meal replacement powder (with beta-glucans from soluble oat fiber) mixed in 12 ounces of water

healthy chocolate chip cookies

***Before Bed***

*Exercise:* Go for a walk outdoors or participate in a favorite sport or recreational activity. During exercise, drink 8 ounces of water.

*Supplements:* Take one serving of a fiber/green superfood combination containing ground flaxseed, mixed in 12 to 16 ounces of water or raw vegetable juice.

*Body therapy:* Take a warm bath, with eight drops of biblical essential oils added, for fifteen minutes.

*Advanced hygiene:* Practice advanced hygiene.

*Sleep:* Go to bed by 10:30 p.m.

# Key #6

## *Avoid Deadly Emotions*

**Nicki:** Do you know the definition of PMS?

Answer: "Permissible Man Slaughter."

When I said in the Introduction that I didn't expect Jordan to fully understand the more sensitive health issues woman face, I was referring to topics like premenstrual syndrome, which many husbands would say is a deadly emotion since their wives get emotional *and* deadly just before the onset of their menstrual flow.

Strange things happen to a woman's body during the premenstrual cycle. Personally, I've battled intense, nonstop cravings for a Starbucks Caramel Macchiato right before the start of my periods. Every four weeks, or so it seemed, deep yearnings for a caramel-flavored coffee drink flooded my consciousness, right on schedule.

After being married to Jordan, I knew that a Starbucks coffee drink wasn't the healthiest beverage out there, but my cravings always won out. Since I viewed myself as health conscious, I thought I was being "good" when I asked the Starbucks *barista* to make mine with organic milk to offset the damage of ordering extra caramel and whipped cream. As you would expect, drinking a Caramel Macchiato never made me feel better or lifted my spirits. In fact, I usually became crankier, and if Jordan happened to be in the vicinity, he certainly picked up the vibe that this was the time of the month not to mess with me.

Jordan was wise not to say anything, but I knew what he thought anyway: *Nicki, drinking a caramel coffee with whipped cream is one of the worst things you could do for your body. You would be better off eating a piece of fruit.*

But I didn't want to hear *that* on the eve of my period. One time, Jordan tsked-tsked me for eating some junk food during my premenstrual time, which prompted a sharp retort from me, but then I heard a little voice in my head repeating Joyce Meyer's advice: "Control your emotions; don't let your emotions control you." My shoulders slumped because I realized I hadn't handled the situation very well.

If you're nodding your head, it's because you're among the three-fourths of women who experience premenstrual symptoms like mood swings, breast tenderness, bloating, and food cravings.[1] Others feel tired or "down," or become irritable. Around 10 percent of menstruating women experience PMS symptoms so severe that it causes drastic mood swings and outbursts of anger, even suicidal thoughts, while interfering with job performance and family relationships.[2]

*The Encyclopedia for Natural Healing* says many PMS symptoms can be linked to an imbalance of prostaglandins, hormonelike fatty acids that affect body processes,[3] but the root causes of PMS have yet to be discovered. At least we're beyond the days when some doctors viewed PMS as some kind of psychological problem. Indeed, there is considerable evidence that PMS has a hormonal basis related to estrogen dominance, which Dr. Wilson talked about in the last chapter.

All I know is that PMS has thrown me for a loop twice in my life. The first time happened when I was a high-school freshman, and I passed out after class, and the other occurred after I was married. I was standing in front of a health food store with Jordan one day while he shot the breeze with the owner. I began seeing stars, but I didn't want to interrupt their conversation and say, "Guys, guess what? I'm really not feeling so good." So I waited . . . and waited . . . and suddenly fainted and collapsed to the ground.

When I came to, Jordan insisted that we go to the hospital—in an ambulance—where an ER doctor poked and prodded before declaring that I had a low heart rate and low blood sugar, probably due to the fact that I was dehydrated. I realized that I had not drunk one ounce that day, and it was 1:00 in the afternoon. I certainly learned the importance of hydration, especially during PMS.

**Jordan:** My recommendation to women with PMS is to eat a lot of cleansing fruits and vegetables. Every juicy fruit is cleansing—watermelon, oranges, grapes, anything citrus. Most vegetables are cleansing, too, and provide lots of water and fiber. This would be a great time to eat more raw foods and less processed foods. I've also heard excellent reports about how exercise reduces PMS symptoms.

On the supplement side, omega-3 cod-liver oil contains essential fatty acids that can help correct hormone imbalance, as does vitamin E. Another vitamin, $B_6$, is known in nutritional circles to be effective for PMS symptoms, especially those associated with high estrogen levels. Tori Hudson, author of *Women's Encyclopedia of Natural Medicine*, reported that magnesium has shown some beneficial effect in the treatment of PMS from women who took the mineral and answered a menstrual distress questionnaire afterward.[4]

The hormonal imbalances intrinsic to PMS are brought about by an intricate set of factors, especially poor nutrition habits: eating too much sugar, salt, coffee, and refined white-flour products. When Nicki drinks Caramel Macchiatos on the eve of her period, the caffeine stimulates her central nervous system, causing anxiousness or irritability. Phyllis Balch, author of *Prescription for Nutritional Healing*, points to studies showing that women who regularly consume caffeine are four times as likely as others to have severe PMS.[5]

But monthly PMS is not the only deadly emotion women must deal with. Anxiety disorders are the most common of emotional disorders and affect more than 25 million Americans, according to the American Psychiatric Association. Anxiety disorders differ from normal feelings of nervousness. Symptom may include:

- overwhelming feelings of panic and fear
- uncontrollable obsessive thoughts
- painful, intrusive memories
- recurring nightmares
- physical symptoms, such as feeling sick to your stomach, heart pounding, and muscle tension.[6]

Women are twice as vulnerable to anxiety disorder and panic attacks than men. Fluctuations in the levels of female hormones and cycles play an important role, but the exact causes of anxiety remain unknown. Those who study anxiety disorders say the affliction can run in families, which suggests that a combination of genes and environmental stresses can produce the disorders. Anxiety disorders are chronic, relentless, and can progressively worsen if not treated. I love the Scripture that speaks directly about what to do with our anxiety, Philippians 4:6–7, which says, "Be anxious for nothing, but in everything by prayer and supplication, with thanksgiving, let your requests be made known to God; and the peace of God, which surpasses all understanding, will guard your hearts and minds through Christ Jesus" (NKJV).

Depression often accompanies anxiety disorders, and when it does, it needs to be treated as well. Symptoms of depression include feelings of sadness, hopelessness, changes in appetite or sleep, low energy, and difficulty concentrating, according to the National Institute of Mental Health. Most people with depression can be effectively treated with antidepressant medications, certain types of psychotherapy, or a combination of both.

Women are twice as likely as men to suffer from depression, a whole-body illness that affects mood, thoughts, and behavior.[7] Depression affects the way you eat and sleep, the way you feel about yourself, and the way you react to people and circumstances around you. Called the common cold of mental illness, depressive disorders affect a staggering 19 million adults in this country.[8]

"Depressed individuals tend to have generally poor health habits, which place them at even higher risk of developing most types of disease," says my friend Don Colbert, MD, and author of *Deadly Emotions.* "The lifestyle choices of the depressed person nearly always result in poor nutrition, little exercise, use of alcohol or drugs, or the overuse of prescription medications. Poor sleep patterns often cause fatigue. The composite result of these bad health habits is a decreased immune function and a greater risk for developing cardiovascular diseases, diabetes, and more frequent infectious diseases."[9]

Like PMS, the causes of depression are not well understood by medicine. Depression episodes can be triggered by tension, stress, a traumatic event, chemical imbalances in the brain, thyroid disorders, nutritional deficiencies, poor diet, the overconsumption of sugar, lack of exercise, and food allergies.[10] As you might tell, depression really is like a downward spiral. Those worried about a lack of sleep often sleep even worse. Those eating a diet heavy in junk foods get depressed because they gain weight and lack energy, which leads to even more bad eating habits, like bingeing.

Although depressed women outnumber depressed men by a two-to-one margin, they are more likely to talk about their problems and reach out for help, and that's a good start. Common treatments for depression are counseling and psychotherapy or taking antidepressant medications like Prozac, Zoloft, and Paxil. The American Psychiatric Society estimates that 80 to 90 percent of the cases of depression could be treated effectively with therapy, though many prefer to receive a prescription for an antidepressant medication.

It is beyond the scope of this book to get into a discussion on antidepressant medications since depression is not easily understood and usually involves some sort of therapy in conjunction with medications. But a *Journal of the American Medical Association* (JAMA) study confirms the insidious sway that drug advertising has upon our culture and how a doctor's diagnosis is not necessarily based on professional judgment but is influenced by patients asking for a specific drug heavily advertised on TV.

In this particular JAMA study,[11] actors pretended to be patients with symptoms of stress and fatigue. They were sent to 152 doctor's offices to see whether they could get prescriptions. Most who did not report symptoms of depression were not given medications, but when they asked for the antidepressant Paxil by name, 55 percent received prescriptions, and 50 percent were diagnosed with clinical depression.[12] Now you know why those bright and cheery TV ads remind you to "ask your doctor about Paxil" or whatever drug they are promoting.

Deadly emotions such as depression and stress alter the chemistry of your body, and unchecked emotions can be a pervasive force in determining your daily behavior. Apathy and helplessness cause a cycle of passivity and helplessness, which further erodes self-confidence. Women, more so than men, seem to emotionally beat themselves up for doing something stupid, saying the wrong thing, or for allowing themselves to gain far more weight than they ever thought possible. Not dealing with emotional issues leads to stress, anger, self-pity, and resentment.

On the other side of the coin, positive emotions, such as laughter, compassion, and love, lift the spirits. "A merry heart doeth good like a medicine," Proverbs 17:22 reminds us (KJV). The next time you feel down, take a walk or make some time for yourself to emotionally turn things around. You might even call a friend who's always upbeat and can make you laugh.

*Spousal Spats Can Damage Your Heart*
*by Jordan Rubin*

Every couple has hot-button issues—finances, in-laws, or vacations—but arguing about them until the cows come home may be a factor in developing coronary atherosclerosis, or hardening of the arteries of the heart. This was confirmed by a University of Utah study of 150 married couples brought into a lab and asked to pick a subject that often triggered fights.

Researchers also found that women who behaved in a hostile manner during marital disputes were more likely to have atherosclerosis, especially if their husbands were also hostile.[13] But husbands who made lots of domineering remarks during arguments also showed an increased risk for heart disease. More ammunition that there is a direct connection between emotions and physical health.

One of the deadliest of all emotions is unforgiveness that turns to bitterness. Are there people in your life who've either done you a great injustice—or bug you so much—that you can't find it in your heart to forgive them? It's a question worth pondering because I believe an unforgiving heart is an underlying factor in many health problems, including chronic, incurable illnesses.

One day, as I sat down for breakfast with Dr. Bruce Wilkinson, author of *The Prayer of Jabez*, our conversation drifted toward people who harbor unforgiveness in their hearts. I'll never forget what Dr. Wilkinson said next: "Jordan, is there anyone in *your* life that you need to forgive?"

The question sounded preposterous. I didn't think I needed to forgive anyone. I thought of myself as a don't-look-back, don't-hold-grudges type of person. I've sped through life with gusto, not as someone who was hung up on something from the past.

"No," I replied. "I don't hold any grudges."

But Dr. Wilkinson wasn't satisfied. "Isn't there *anyone* in your life you need to forgive?"

You know how when someone asks you, "How are you?" twice in the same conversation, he or she wants to know how you are *really* doing? That's what Dr. Wilkinson did that morning, so I stopped and reflected for a moment. *Were* there people I needed to forgive? The more I thought about it . . . "Yes, there have been some people who have hurt me," I confided, "but I've moved on. I've forgiven them."

There—a chink in my armor. Dr. Wilkinson called me on it. "I don't believe you," he declared.

He was right. I was only fooling myself if I thought I had really forgiven those who'd hurt me in the past.

"What do I have to do to forgive someone?" I asked.

"A great way to forgive somebody is to take a white sheet of paper or a pad and write down the name of the person you need to forgive at the top," Dr. Wilkinson began. "Ask the Lord to show you grievances that person has caused you, and then write down the things that person did to cause you pain."

"Then what?"

"Then you ask God to cleanse you of your past unforgiveness. By the time you've reached this step, you'll be heading down the road to recovery. After you've completed your list, which may take up several sheets, write down the following: *Lord, help me love*—insert the person's name here—*the way You love him.* After that, you should tear up the paper or burn it."

I thanked Dr. Wilkinson for his advice, and our breakfast discussion turned to other topics. Later, when I had a private moment, I sat down with a piece of paper and thought about people whom I had never forgiven. I recalled doctors who told me in the midst of my health challenges that my illness was my fault. There were relatives and friends who said they would visit me in the hospital when I was deathly ill, but they never came. There were people who, for no apparent reason, tried to thwart my efforts to help God's people get healthy, and those who had taken advantage of me in business.

I wrote each name on a piece of paper and stared at it, thinking back to what each one did to cause such bitterness in my heart. Then I bowed my head and asked God to help me forgive these people just as He forgave me for my past sins. When I was through making peace with the Lord, I ripped the paper into pieces and tossed it into the wastebasket of history.

Harboring unforgiveness that turns to bitterness is like drinking poison and expecting the person who hurt you to die. And worst of all, unforgiveness is a sin. Jesus said, "For if you forgive men their trespasses, your heavenly Father will also forgive you. But if you do not forgive men their trespasses, neither will your Father forgive your trespasses" (Matt. 6:14–15 NKJV).

After speaking at a church in Kansas City, Missouri, and talking about the Seven Keys, including the importance of forgiving others, I met a remarkable woman named Gidget Stous from Oak Grove, Missouri, twenty-eight miles east of Kansas City. She stood in line to have a word with me, and when we met, she described a remarkable story about her health transformation and about how she had to forgive her ex-husband who left her for another woman, as well as those who had made mean, cutting remarks about her weight gain following the birth of her children.

Gidget gave me permission to relate her story, which began when she married at age seventeen and reached a crisis point after her divorce when she became a single-parent mom to two preteen children. The stress of raising kids on her own and owning an insurance agency came crashing on her shoulders that Christmas. She reacted to the anxiety by snacking on Christmas cookies left at the office, eating every scrap of delicious food on her plate when she lunched with the "girls," and not denying herself at the holiday buffet tables. When Gidget finally gathered up the courage to look in a mirror, the sight of a twenty-seven-year-old woman who had let herself go horrified her.

She reluctantly stepped on the scale and gasped at her weight: 230 pounds. What a mess her life had become! Her doctor pronounced her a borderline diabetic—type 2—and diagnosed her with a case of adult ADHD, prompting him to prescribe a pair of strong medications—Paxil and Adderall. She quickly became addicted to both drugs. Her chart revealed other afflictions: acid reflux, allergies, hypertension, elevated cholesterol levels, and endometriosis.

"I had really low energy, was miserable, and terribly stressed about everything happening in my life," she told me. Things began to turn around when she began dating a fellow named Mike. Her boyfriend gave her one of my earlier books, *The Maker's Diet*, but she put the book aside for several months until she finally began reading it one evening.

When she came to the section on why I don't eat pork (because God didn't design our bodies to eat scavenger animals), Gidget's immediate reaction was, "No way." She had an emotional attachment to bacon on her breakfast plate and pork chops with mashed potatoes and gravy for dinner. That was how she was raised. But as she took stock, she remembered what her doctor had said during her last visit: "Gidget, you have the cholesterol level of a sixty-five-year-old woman. If you don't do something soon, you won't see your children grow up."

After she married Mike, she took the Bible's health advice to heart and realized immediate results. She adopted the advanced hygiene program outlined in Key #3 and said the morning and evening facial dips took care of her allergies. She exchanged the half dozen Cokes she drank at her desk for bottled water. She stopped eating processed foods and unclean meats. She, Mike, and her children even volunteered to do chores at a nearby farm in exchange for raw milk, free-range eggs, real butter, and grass-fed beef and chicken.

In less than six months, she lost eighty-five pounds. "Many of my longtime customers at the office didn't recognize me when I got down to 140 pounds. After the extra weight went away, so did my stress," Gidget told me. There was another deadly emotion, however, that Gidget had to deal with, and it was unforgiveness.

Her failed marriage had devastated her self-esteem. After she added weight following the birth of her children, acquaintances made subtle digs: "Are you really going to eat that?" or "Have you thought about trying this diet?"

"These women were the most insensitive to me," Gidget said. "They'd make these little remarks while they were eating the same junk at lunch."

Gidget did exactly what I learned from Bruce Wilkinson about dealing with unforgiveness in your heart. She wrote down the name of her ex-husband as well as those who had made cutting remarks about her weight and appearance over the years. Next to each name she listed each grievance she had against them. Then she asked God to help her forgive them, crumpled up the paper, and tossed it into the trash. "I had issues with people who were mean to me, including family members," Gidget said. "One way or another, I had to forgive them because otherwise I'd become too stressed over the whole thing."

I love Gidget's story, but what about you? If you're still annoyed by those who teased you about your body shape, made snide comments about your plus-size clothes, or told you that you'll never lose weight, you have to let it go. Sure, words can hurt, and words can break a heart. But even though your "friends" were mean to you, that's history. Deborah Newman, author of *A Woman's Search for Worth,* said that before she ever forgave others or helped individuals learn to forgive, she also thought forgiveness granted all the benefits to the offender. In the process of dealing with forgiveness, she found that it was her own soul that received the greatest benefit from forgiving others.

Forgiveness has positive physical benefits as well. Your health will always take a hit if you're harboring resentment in your heart, nursing a grudge into overtime, or plotting revenge against those who hurt you. High levels of anger may help drive coronary heart disease, according to a study reported in the *Mayo Clinic Proceedings.*[14] Bottling up deadly emotions such as anger, bitterness, and resentment will produce toxins similar to bingeing on a dozen glazed doughnuts. The efficiency of your immune system decreases noticeably for six hours when you're anxious and fearful, and staying angry and bitter about those who have teased you in the past can alter the chemistry of your body—

and even prompt you to fall off the healthy food wagon. An old proverb states it well: "What you are eating is not nearly as important as what's eating you."

It should come as no surprise to you what a major role negative emotions play in your body's healing processes. Dr. Joe Mercola, writing on his popular Web site, www.mercola.com, said the connection between your mind and your body is strong and well documented by a mountain of scientific research. "That's why healing your mind is a crucial step in keeping your body healthy," he wrote.[15]

I began speaking at Women of Faith weekend conference events in 2006, and I've enjoyed getting to know Patsy Clairmont, who, at one time, suffered for years as a prisoner in her home, a victim of agoraphobia, or fear of open spaces.

She was just out of high school when she married Les and moved from Michigan to Louisville, Kentucky, where Les had joined the Army as a mechanic. A couple of years into their marriage, when Patsy was in her early twenties, Les noticed that she never—well, almost never—left the apartment. When he inquired why, Patsy told Les that she was afraid to go to the grocery store because the aisles seemed to swallow her up. Then he noticed that she listened to weather reports all day long and would hide under the dining room table whenever thunderstorms struck her neighborhood.

Patsy knew something wasn't right when she experienced panic attacks, especially when she became angry. One attack occurred at home; her windpipes fought for air, and Patsy staggered around the living room until a concerned Les rushed her to the emergency room. A shot of Demerol knocked her out and ended the panic attack.

Patsy said it took her years to take personal responsibility for a lifestyle that had evolved into an around-the-clock existence of gulping tranquilizers, smoking two packs of cigarettes, and drinking fifteen to twenty cups of coffee each day. When subsequent panic attacks landed her in the hospital again, she met another patient, Mary Ann Tanner, while walking about the hospital. They struck up a conversation, and Mary Ann invited Patsy to attend a women's weekend retreat. Patsy was a believer but didn't know how to function as one.

At this low moment in her life, she felt she needed Christ so much that she was willing to risk leaving her house to attend the retreat.

As she left for the conference, Les bade his wife good-bye and wondered when he would receive a phone call asking to pick her up. But Patsy persevered and stayed for the entire conference.

The reason Patsy eagerly remained was because she learned about Jesus with those loving women—that Jesus had the power to change her internally and externally. She learned how to apply the salve of God's Word to her troubled life, and that's something you can do too, because Jesus has the power to change you inside and out.

Patsy's transformation was total, and the person most impressed with the changes was the person who knew her best: Les. He witnessed a year of spiritual growth before he, too, decided that what he needed was Jesus Christ in his life. He and Patsy knelt in their living room when he gave his heart to Christ.

"When a person changes," says Patsy, "it takes time for those around her to adjust and figure out what that means to their relationship. We complicate the adjustment to our change when we insist on trying to take everyone with us. Truth is, we can't change other people; only God can do that. We can, though, extend grace to them. Grace is the space that allows others to grow or not grow, to agree or disagree, to change or remain unchanged. No wonder grace is a gift from God; left on our own, we humans just don't have that kind of spacious room inside us."[16]

In years past, Patsy has taken the Women of Faith stage with an interesting prop—a footlong braid of hundreds of colored rubber bands. "These rubber bands represent my tangled emotions and everything I have to deal with," she explained one time. Patsy said her lonely journey gave her a deep appreciation of God's healing power as He pulled together the emotionally fragmented pieces of her life. "My life illustrates that imperfect, 'cracked' Christians are God's specialty," she said.

Life will never be perfect, and stuff happens. If you follow the *Great Physician's Rx for Women's Health*, I'm not promising a bed of roses, but I'm confident that allowing God's healing power in your life will help you deal with any deadly emotions weighing on your mind. Please remember that no matter how badly you've been hurt in the past, it's still possible to forgive. So forgive those who've hurt you, and then let it go because life really is too short. "We are all here for a spell; get all the good laughs you can," humorist Will Rogers once said.

*Postpartum Blues*
*by Nicki Rubin*

There's no doubt that childbirth is an emotionally intense event, but after I brought Joshua home from the hospital, I experienced a minor case of the "baby blues," a fairly common experience for 80 percent of new moms. Doctors characterize the baby blues as crying spells, mood swings, and irritability beginning three days after birth and resolving on its own in two weeks.

Women who don't get over the baby blues after a couple of weeks usually go on to develop postpartum depression, which happens to more than 10 percent of new moms.[17] They may experience a sense of being overwhelmed, an inability to sleep, or poor appetite.

Doctors say postpartum depression is caused by hormonal shifts that happen after childbirth when a woman's levels of estrogen and progesterone rapidly fall to nonpregnant levels. The change in hormone levels prompts reactions from sleeplessness to irritability, mental confusion, and even psychosis.

Actress Brooke Shields went public with her battle with postpartum depression following the birth of her daughter, Rowan Francis, in 2003. She said her baby seemed like a stranger to her; she dreaded the moments her husband brought Rowan to her, and she couldn't bear the sound of her daughter crying. At her lowest point, Brooke thought about jumping out of her apartment window. Without antidepressant medications and weekly therapy sessions, Brooke said her life would have been a mess.

From talking with friends, I know that postpartum depression is real, which is why it's critical to young mothers to cry out for help, seek counseling, and talk with their doctors.

As for myself, I mitigated the baby blues by eating as naturally as I could before Joshua's birth, taking supplements, practicing advanced hygiene so I wouldn't get sick, and remaining as active as my body would allow.

### *What Women Are Saying*
### *by Angela Roysdon*

I'll never forget the time when I was eighteen years old and lying in bed one night, praying for God to mold and shape me, when flashbulb memories started to break loose—memories of molestation.

Shortly after that, I drifted away from my walk with the Lord and ended up in the throes of deep depression. I tried everything to fill the void—everything except coming back to the Lord. Before I knew it, I was pregnant and marrying a man who would become very abusive to me and our two children. By my third anniversary, I was in a safe house, where I was served with divorce papers.

The children and I went to live with my parents, who helped me realize that I needed the Lord. I started attending church regularly again and felt myself growing closer to God. Then I would hit a brick wall and struggle.

I enrolled in a "Change of Heart" class at church, which helped me forgive the seventeen-year-old boy who had done some terrible things to me. Since the molestation, I had always struggled with my weight, topping the chart at 320 pounds. I thought about having gastric bypass surgery.

In September 2004, I met a man with two children the same ages as my daughter, Hunter, and son, Logan. Jason and I became friends and were married in December 2005. Shortly before we were married, we were at a dinner party with some friends and my niece, who is only nine months younger than me. She asked to have a private conversation with me.

We walked over to a corner of the living room, where she told me about repressed memories about a boy who had molested her—the same boy who had taken advantage of me at a small church in North Carolina. Many of the things I had repressed came up again to my memory as I listened to my niece tell her story. My mind was screaming, *Oh, God, I've been raped.* Some of the things that were done were gruesome. For instance, my ob-gyn had asked me about scars on my cervix when my daughter was born, but I had no idea where they came from.

When we left the dinner party, I told Jason about my conversation with my niece. About halfway into it, he said he couldn't take it anymore. "I love you and support you 150 percent, and I will be at your side through all this, but we need to find someone for you to talk to."

That night, more memories came back to mind. I remember lying on my Sunday school room floor while I was being raped, looking up to the picture of Jesus, silently begging Him to help me. *Please, Jesus, make him stop.*

I received more counseling and prayer for deliverance. I forgave my tormentor again. Some time later, Jordan Rubin came to our church, and I told Jason afterward that I wanted to take the 7 Weeks of Wellness challenge that our church was going through. This 49-day program was based on the Great Physician's Rx.

I started losing weight immediately. I felt so much healthier and had more energy. When we got to the sixth week and Key #6, "Avoid Deadly Emotions," I prayed, *God, have I forgiven everyone?*

I kept hearing a voice saying, *No, not everyone.*

Kelli Williams was our teacher that evening, and she told us that she had been put on bed rest days before her wedding, which threw her for a loop. She said her mother came by to see her and asked her if she had forgiven God. That's when I felt my breath catch in my throat.

*God, am I mad at You?* I asked. The Lord brought back memories of the rape and looking up at the picture of Jesus. He spoke to my spirit and said, *I love you, and I have never wanted anything bad for you.*

"God, I am so sorry," I prayed. "I've held this against You." As I wept, I felt a mental weight melt off me. I felt free and happy for the first time in many, many years.

*The Great Physician's Rx for Women's Health* is much more than a diet. It is a life-changing health plan that will transform your body, mind, and spirit. I know firsthand because these principles changed my life.

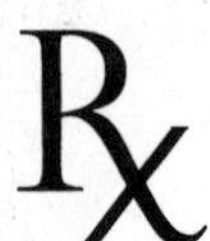

## THE GREAT PHYSICIAN'S Rx FOR WOMEN'S HEALTH: AVOID DEADLY EMOTIONS

- *Do your best to avoid stress, anxiety, fear, and anger.*
- *Realize that you're susceptible to getting sick when you're sad, scared, or stressed by everyday life.*
- *Trust God when you face circumstances that cause you to worry or become anxious.*
- *Practice forgiveness every day, and forgive those that hurt you.*

### THE GREAT PHYSICIAN'S RX FOR WEEK #6

Remember to visit www.BiblicalHealthInstitute.com and click on the GPRx Resource Guide for recommended food, nutritional supplement, advanced hygiene, exercise and body therapy, air and water purification, and skin and body care products.

### DAY 36

*You will notice that some items in the meal plans that follow are italicized. You can find the recipes for these—and over other 250 delicious and healthy recipes—at www.BiblicalHealthInstitute.com.*

*Upon Waking*

*Advanced hygiene:* Practice advanced hygiene.

*Reduce toxins:* Open windows for one hour today. Use natural soap, skin and body care products, facial care products, toothpaste, and hair care products.

*Supplements:* Take one serving of a fiber/green superfood combination containing ground flaxseed, mixed in 12 to 16 ounces of water or raw vegetable juice.

*Body therapy:* Get twenty minutes of direct sunlight.

*Exercise:* Perform functional fitness exercises for fifteen minutes, or spend fifteen minutes on the rebounder. Finish with ten minutes of deep-breathing exercises. During exercise, drink 8 ounces of water.

*Emotional health:* When you face a circumstance that would usually cause you to worry, repeat the following: "Lord, I trust You. I cast my cares upon You, and I believe that You're going to take care of [insert your current situation]." Confess that throughout the day, whenever you think about your circumstance.

*Breakfast*

Drink 8 ounces of water during breakfast.

two eggs (omega-3 or organic, and prepared as desired)

one piece of fruit

one piece of whole grain sprouted or sourdough toast with butter

hot tea with honey

*Supplements:* Take two whole food multivitamin caplets, one capsule of omega-3 cod-liver oil, and two caplets of a whole food calcium/magnesium blend.

*Between Breakfast and Lunch*

Drink 12 ounces of water.

*Lunch*

During lunch, drink 8 ounces of water.

green salad with 3 ounces of chicken and carrots, red onions, cucumbers, and yellow peppers

healthy salad dressing with one tablespoon of extra-virgin olive oil or high-lignan flaxseed oil

one piece of fruit

*Supplements:* Take two whole food multivitamin caplets, one capsule of omega-3 cod-liver oil, and two caplets of a whole food calcium/magnesium blend.

***Between Lunch and Dinner***

Drink 12 ounces of water.

***Dinner***

During dinner, drink 8 ounces of water

fish of choice

brown rice

grilled asparagus

green salad with red or yellow peppers, red onions, green or red cabbage, celery, cucumbers, and carrots

healthy salad dressing with olive oil and/or high-lignan flaxseed oil

*Supplements:* Take two whole food multivitamin caplets, one capsule of omega-3 cod-liver oil, and two caplets of a whole food calcium/magnesium blend.

***Snack/Dessert***

apple cinnamon whole food bar (with beta-glucans from soluble oat fiber)

whole-milk yogurt, fruit, and honey

***Before Bed***

*Exercise:* Go for a walk outdoors or participate in a favorite sport or recreational activity. During exercise, drink 8 ounces of water.

*Supplements:* Take one serving of a fiber/green superfood combination containing ground flaxseed, mixed in 12 to 16 ounces of water or raw vegetable juice.

*Body therapy:* Take a warm bath, with eight drops of biblical essential oils added, for fifteen minutes.

*Advanced hygiene:* Practice advanced hygiene.

*Sleep:* Go to bed by 10:30 p.m.

## Day 37

*You will notice that some items in the meal plans that follow are italicized. You can find the recipes for these—and over other 250 delicious and healthy recipes—at www.BiblicalHealthInstitute.com.*

### *Upon Waking*

*Advanced hygiene:* Practice advanced hygiene. See page 277 for guidance.

*Reduce toxins:* Open windows for one hour today. Use natural soap, skin and body care products, facial care products, toothpaste, and hair care products.

*Supplements:* Take one serving of a fiber/green superfood combination containing ground flaxseed, mixed in 12 to 16 ounces of water or raw vegetable juice.

*Exercise:* Perform functional fitness exercises for fifteen minutes, or spend fifteen minutes on the rebounder. Finish with ten minutes of deep-breathing exercises. During exercise, drink 8 ounces of water.

*Body therapy:* Take a hot-and-cold shower.

*Emotional health:* When you face a circumstance that would usually cause you to worry, repeat the following: "Lord, I trust You. I cast my cares upon You, and I believe that You're going to take care of [insert your current situation]." Confess that throughout the day, whenever you think about your circumstance.

### *Breakfast*

During breakfast, drink 8 ounces of water.

For a healthy smoothie, mix the following in a blender:

8 ounces plain whole milk, yogurt, or kefir

1 tablespoon honey

1/2 cup fresh or frozen fruit (bananas, peaches, berries, pineapple, etc.)

1 teaspoon high-lignan flaxseed oil

1 serving of protein powder (optional)

*Supplements:* Take two whole food multivitamin caplets, one capsule of omega-3 cod-liver oil, and two caplets of a whole food calcium/magnesium blend.

*Between Breakfast and Lunch*

Drink 12 ounces of water.

*Lunch*

During lunch, drink 8 ounces of water.

low-mercury, high omega-3 tuna on sprouted or yeast-free whole-grain bread with lettuce, tomato, and sprouts

one piece of fruit

*Supplements:* Take two whole food multivitamin caplets, one capsule of omega-3 cod-liver oil, and two caplets of a whole food calcium/magnesium blend.

*Between Lunch and Dinner*

Drink 12 ounces of water.

*Dinner*

During dinner, drink 8 ounces of water.

chicken of choice

quinoa with onions

green salad with red or yellow peppers, red onions, green or red cabbage, celery, cucumbers, and carrots

healthy salad dressing with olive oil and/or high-lignan flaxseed oil

*Supplements:* Take two whole food multivitamin caplets, one capsule of omega-3 cod-liver oil, and two caplets of a whole food calcium/magnesium blend.

*Snack/Dessert*

whole food meal replacement powder (with beta-glucans from soluble oat fiber) mixed in 12 ounces of water

cottage cheese, honey, and berries

*Before Bed*

*Exercise:* Go for a walk outdoors or participate in a favorite sport or recreational activity. During exercise, drink 8 ounces of water.

*Supplements:* Take one serving of a fiber/green superfood combination containing ground flaxseed, mixed in 12 to 16 ounces of water or raw vegetable juice.

*Advanced hygiene:* Practice advanced hygiene.

*Emotional health:* Ask the Lord to bring to your mind someone you need to forgive. Take out a sheet of paper and write the person's name at the top. Try to remember each specific action that person did against you that brought you pain. Write down the following: "I forgive [insert person's name] for [insert the action he or she did against you]." After you fill up the paper, tear it up or burn it, and ask God to give you the strength to truly forgive that person.

*Body therapy:* Spend ten minutes listening to soothing music before retiring.

*Sleep:* Go to bed by 10:30 p.m.

## DAY 38

*You will notice that some items in the meal plans that follow are italicized. You can find the recipes for these—and over other 250 delicious and healthy recipes—at www.BiblicalHealthInstitute.com.*

### *Upon Waking*

*Advanced hygiene:* Practice advanced hygiene. See page 277 for guidance.

*Reduce toxins:* Open windows for one hour today. Use natural soap, skin and body care products, facial care products, toothpaste, and hair care products.

*Supplements:* Take one serving of a fiber/green superfood combination containing ground flaxseed, mixed in 12 to 16 ounces of water or raw vegetable juice.

*Exercise:* Perform functional fitness exercises for fifteen minutes, or spend fifteen minutes on the rebounder. Finish with ten minutes of deep-breathing exercises. During exercise, drink 8 ounces of water.

*Body therapy:* Get twenty minutes of direct sunlight.

*Emotional health:* When you face a circumstance that would usually cause you to worry, repeat the following: "Lord, I trust You. I cast my cares upon You, and I believe that You're going to take care of [insert your current situation]." Confess that throughout the day, whenever you think about your circumstance.

*Breakfast*

During breakfast, drink 8 ounces of water.

sprouted dry cereal with yogurt, goat's milk, or almond milk

banana

hot tea with honey

*Supplements:* Take two whole food multivitamin caplets, one capsule of omega-3 cod-liver oil, and two caplets of a whole food calcium/magnesium blend.

*Between Breakfast and Lunch*

Drink 12 ounces of water.

*Lunch*

During lunch, drink 8 ounces of water.

green salad with 3 ounces of steak and carrots, red onions, cucumbers, and yellow peppers

healthy salad dressing with one tablespoon of extra-virgin olive oil or high-lignan flaxseed oil

one piece of fruit

*Supplements:* Take two whole food multivitamin caplets, one capsule of omega-3 cod-liver oil, and two caplets of a whole food calcium/magnesium blend.

*Between Lunch and Dinner*

Drink 12 ounces of water.

*Dinner*

During dinner, drink 8 ounces of water.

red meat of choice

peas and carrots

green salad with red or yellow peppers, red onions, green or red cabbage, celery, cucumbers, and carrots

healthy salad dressing with olive oil and/or high-lignan flaxseed oil

*Supplements:* Take two whole food multivitamin caplets, one capsule of omega-3 cod-liver oil, and two caplets of a whole food calcium/magnesium blend.

*Snack/Dessert*

berry antioxidant whole food bar (with beta-glucans from soluble oat fiber)

apple with almond or sesame butter (tahini)

*Before Bed*

*Exercise:* Go for a walk outdoors or participate in a favorite sport or recreational activity. During exercise, drink 8 ounces of water.

*Supplements:* Take one serving of a fiber/green superfood combination containing ground flaxseed, mixed in 12 to 16 ounces of water or raw vegetable juice.

*Advanced hygiene:* Practice advanced hygiene.

*Emotional health:* Ask the Lord to bring to your mind someone you need to forgive. Take out a sheet of paper and write the person's name at the top. Try to remember each specific action that person did against you that brought you pain. Write down the following: "I forgive [insert person's name] for [insert the action he or she did against you]." After you fill up the paper, tear it up or burn it, and ask God to give you the strength to truly forgive that person.

*Body therapy:* Take a warm bath, with eight drops of biblical essential oils added, for fifteen minutes.

*Sleep:* Go to bed by 10:30 p.m.

## DAY 39

*You will notice that some items in the meal plans that follow are italicized. You can find the recipes for these—and over other 250 delicious and healthy recipes—at www.BiblicalHealthInstitute.com.*

*Upon Waking*

*Advanced hygiene:* Practice advanced hygiene. See page 277 for guidance.

*Reduce toxins:* Open windows for one hour today. Use natural soap, skin and body care products, facial care products, toothpaste, and hair care products.

*Supplements:* Take one serving of a fiber/green superfood combination containing ground flaxseed, mixed in 12 to 16 ounces of water or raw vegetable juice.

*Exercise:* Perform functional fitness exercises for fifteen minutes, or spend fifteen minutes on the rebounder. Finish with ten minutes of deep-breathing exercises. During exercise, drink 8 ounces of water.

*Body therapy:* Take a hot-and-cold shower.

*Emotional health:* When you face a circumstance that would usually cause you to worry, repeat the following: "Lord, I trust You. I cast my cares upon You, and I believe that You're going to take care of [insert your current situation]." Confess that throughout the day, whenever you think about your circumstance.

***Breakfast***

During breakfast, drink 8 ounces of water.

For a healthy smoothie, mix the following in a blender:

8 ounces plain whole milk, yogurt, or kefir

1 tablespoon honey

1/2 cup fresh or frozen fruit (bananas, peaches, berries, pineapple, etc.)

1 teaspoon high-lignan flaxseed oil

1 serving of protein powder (optional)

*Supplements:* Take two whole food multivitamin caplets, one capsule of omega-3 cod-liver oil, and two caplets of a whole food calcium/magnesium blend.

***Between Breakfast and Lunch***

Drink 12 ounces of water.

***Lunch***

During lunch, drink 8 ounces of water.

turkey on sprouted or yeast-free whole-grain bread with lettuce, tomato, and sprouts

one piece of fruit

*Supplements:* Take two whole food multivitamin caplets, one capsule of omega-3 cod-liver oil, and two caplets of a whole food calcium/magnesium blend.

***Between Lunch and Dinner***

Drink 12 ounces of water.

***Dinner***

During dinner, drink 8 ounces of water.

roasted free-range chicken

steamed broccoli

sweet potato

*Supplements:* Take two whole food multivitamin caplets, one capsule of omega-3 cod-liver oil, and two caplets of a whole food calcium/magnesium blend.

***Snack/Dessert***

whole food meal replacement powder (with beta-glucans from soluble oat fiber) mixed in 12 ounces of water

raw veggies with hummus, salsa, and guacamole

***Before Bed***

*Exercise:* Go for a walk outdoors or participate in a favorite sport or recreational activity. During exercise, drink 8 ounces of water.

*Supplements:* Take one serving of a fiber/green superfood combination containing ground flaxseed, mixed in 12 to 16 ounces of water or raw vegetable juice.

*Advanced hygiene*: Practice advanced hygiene.

*Emotional health:* Ask the Lord to bring to your mind someone you need to forgive. Take out a sheet of paper and write the person's name at the top. Try to remember each specific action that person did against you that brought you pain. Write down the following: "I forgive [insert person's name] for [insert the action he or she did against you]." After you fill up the paper, tear it up or burn it, and ask God to give you the strength to truly forgive that person.

*Body therapy:* Spend ten minutes listening to soothing music before you retire.

*Sleep:* Go to bed by 10:30 p.m.

## DAY 40 (PARTIAL-FAST DAY)

*You will notice that some items in the meal plans that follow are italicized. You can find the recipes for these—and over other 250 delicious and healthy recipes—at www.BiblicalHealthInstitute.com.*

***Upon Waking***

*Advanced hygiene:* Practice advanced hygiene. See page 277 for guidance.

*Reduce toxins:* Open windows for one hour today. Use natural soap, skin and body care products, facial care products, toothpaste, and hair care products.

*Supplements:* Take one serving of a fiber/green superfood combination containing ground flaxseed, mixed in 12 to 16 ounces of water or raw vegetable juice.

*Exercise:* Perform functional fitness exercises for fifteen minutes, or spend fifteen minutes on the rebounder. Finish with ten minutes of deep-breathing exercises. During exercise, drink 8 ounces of water.

*Body therapy:* Get twenty minutes of direct sunlight.

*Emotional health:* When you face a circumstance that would usually cause you to worry, repeat the following: "Lord, I trust You. I cast my cares upon You, and I believe that You're going to take care of [insert your current situation]." Confess that throughout the day, whenever you think about your circumstance.

***Breakfast***

none (partial-fast day)

Drink 12 ounces of water.

***Between Breakfast and Lunch***

Drink 12 ounces of water.

***Lunch***

none (partial-fast day)

Drink 12 ounces of water.

***Between Lunch and Dinner***

Drink 12 ounces of water.

***Dinner***

During dinner, drink 8 ounces of water.

*Chicken Soup*

cultured vegetables

green salad with red or yellow peppers, red onions, green or red cabbage, celery, cucumbers, and carrots

healthy salad dressing with olive oil and/or high-lignan flaxseed oil

*Supplements:* Take two whole food multivitamin caplets, one capsule of omega-3 cod-liver oil, and two caplets of a whole food calcium/magnesium blend.

***Snack/Dessert***

none (partial-fast day)

Drink 12 ounces of water.

***Before Bed***

*Exercise:* Go for a walk outdoors or participate in a favorite sport or recreational activity. During exercise, drink 8 ounces of water.

*Supplements:* Take one serving of a fiber/green superfood combination containing ground flaxseed, mixed in 12 to 16 ounces of water or raw vegetable juice.

*Advanced hygiene:* Practice advanced hygiene.

*Emotional health:* Ask the Lord to bring to your mind someone you need to forgive. Take out a sheet of paper and write the person's name at the top. Try to remember each specific action that person did against you that brought you pain. Write down the following: "I forgive [insert person's name] for [insert the action he or she did against you]." After you fill up the paper, tear it up or burn it, and ask God to give you the strength to truly forgive that person.

*Body therapy:* Take a warm bath, with eight drops of biblical essential oils added, for fifteen minutes.

*Sleep:* Go to bed by 10:30 p.m.

## DAY 41 (DAY OF REST)

*You will notice that some items in the meal plans that follow are italicized. You can find the recipes for these—and over other 250 delicious and healthy recipes—at www.BiblicalHealthInstitute.com.*

***Upon Waking***

*Advanced hygiene:* Practice advanced hygiene.

*Reduce toxins:* Open windows for one hour today. Use natural soap, skin and body care products, facial care products, toothpaste, and hair care products.

*Supplements:* Take one serving of a fiber/green superfood combination containing ground flaxseed, mixed in 12 to 16 ounces of water or raw vegetable juice.

*Exercise:* None.

*Body therapies:* None.

*Emotional health:* When you face a circumstance that would usually cause you to worry, repeat the following: "Lord, I trust You. I cast my cares upon You, and I believe that You're going to take care of [insert your current situation]." Confess that throughout the day whenever you think about your circumstance.

***Breakfast***

During breakfast, drink 8 ounces of water.

one whole-grain pancake with maple syrup and butter

4 ounces of whole-milk yogurt with berries and honey and 1/2 teaspoon of high-lignan flaxseed oil (optional)

organic fresh-ground coffee with organic cream and honey

*Supplements:* Take two whole food multivitamin caplets, one capsule of omega-3 cod-liver oil, and two caplets of a whole food calcium/magnesium blend.

***Between Breakfast and Lunch***

Drink 12 ounces of water.

***Lunch***

During lunch, drink 8 ounces of water.

green salad with raw cheese, avocado, walnuts, olives, carrots, red onions, cucumbers, and yellow peppers

healthy salad dressing with one tablespoon of extra-virgin olive oil or high-lignan flaxseed oil

one piece of fruit

*Supplements:* Take two whole food multivitamin caplets, one capsule of omega-3 cod-liver oil, and two caplets of a whole food calcium/magnesium blend.

***Between Lunch and Dinner***

Drink 12 ounces of water.

***Dinner***

During dinner, drink 8 ounces of water.

*Thai Coconut Soup*

baked salmon

*Easy Sautéed Greens*

green salad with red or yellow peppers, red onions, green or red cabbage, celery, cucumbers, and carrots

healthy salad dressing with olive oil and/or high-lignan flaxseed oil

*Supplements:* Take two whole food multivitamin caplets, one capsule of omega-3 cod-liver oil, and two caplets of a whole food calcium/magnesium blend.

***Snack/Dessert***

green superfood whole food bar (with beta-glucans from soluble oat fiber)

*Zesty Popcorn* with butter and spices

***Before Bed***

*Exercise:* Go for a walk outdoors or participate in a favorite sport or recreational activity. During exercise, drink 8 ounces of water.

*Supplements:* Take one serving of a fiber/green superfood combination containing ground flaxseed, mixed in 12 to 16 ounces of water or raw vegetable juice.

*Advanced hygiene:* Practice advanced hygiene.

*Emotional health:* Ask the Lord to bring to your mind someone you need to forgive. Take out a sheet of paper and write the person's name at the top. Try to remember each specific action that person did against you that brought you pain. Write down the following: "I forgive [insert person's name] for [insert the action he or she did against you]." After you fill up the paper, tear it up or burn it, and ask God to give you the strength to truly forgive that person.

*Body therapy:* Spend ten minutes listening to soothing music before you retire.

*Sleep:* Go to bed by 10:30 p.m.

## DAY 42

*You will notice that some items in the meal plans that follow are italicized. You can find the recipes for these—and over other 250 delicious and healthy recipes—at www.BiblicalHealthInstitute.com.*

***Upon Waking***

*Advanced hygiene:* Practice advanced hygiene. See page 277 for guidance.

*Reduce toxins:* Open windows for one hour today. Use natural soap, skin and body care products, facial care products, toothpaste, and hair care products.

*Supplements:* Take one serving of a fiber/green superfood combination containing ground flaxseed, mixed in 12 to 16 ounces of water or raw vegetable juice.

*Exercise:* Perform functional fitness exercises for fifteen minutes, or spend fifteen minutes on the rebounder. Finish with ten minutes of deep-breathing exercises. During exercise, drink 8 ounces of water.

*Body therapy:* Get twenty minutes of direct sunlight.

*Emotional health:* When you face a circumstance that would usually cause you to worry, repeat the following: "Lord, I trust You. I cast my cares upon You, and I believe that You're going to take care of [insert your current situation]." Confess that throughout the day, whenever you think about your circumstance.

***Breakfast***

During breakfast, drink 8 ounces of water.

two-egg omelet with avocado, cheese, tomato, onion, and pepper

*Sautéed Veggies*

hot tea and honey

*Supplements*: Take two whole food multivitamin caplets, one capsule of omega-3 cod-liver oil, and two caplets of a whole food calcium/magnesium blend.

***Between Breakfast and Lunch***

Drink 12 ounces of water.

***Lunch***

During lunch, drink 8 ounces of water.

almond butter and honey or pure fruit jam on sprouted or yeast-free whole-grain bread

one piece of fruit

*Supplements:* Take two whole food multivitamin caplets, one capsule of omega-3 cod-liver oil, and two caplets of a whole food calcium/magnesium blend.

***Between Lunch and Dinner***

Drink 12 ounces of water.

***Dinner***

During dinner, drink 8 ounces of water.

fish of choice

baked potato

green beans

*Supplements:* Take two whole food multivitamin caplets, one capsule of omega-3 cod-liver oil, and two caplets of a whole food calcium/magnesium blend.

*Snack/Dessert*

whole food meal replacement powder (with beta-glucans from soluble oat fiber) mixed in 12 ounces of water

healthy chocolate mousse

*Before Bed*

Drink 8–12 ounces of water or hot tea with honey.

*Exercise:* Go for a walk outdoors or participate in a favorite sport or recreational activity. During exercise, drink 8 ounces of water.

*Supplements:* Take one serving of a fiber/green superfood combination containing ground flaxseed, mixed in 12 to 16 ounces of water or raw vegetable juice.

*Advanced hygiene:* Practice advanced hygiene.

*Emotional health:* Ask the Lord to bring to your mind someone you need to forgive. Take out a sheet of paper and write the person's name at the top. Try to remember each specific action that person did against you that brought you pain. Write down the following: "I forgive [insert person's name] for [insert the action he or she did against you]." After you fill up the paper, tear it up or burn it, and ask God to give you the strength to truly forgive that person.

*Body therapy:* Take a warm bath, with eight drops of biblical essential oils added, for fifteen minutes.

*Sleep:* Go to bed by 10:30 p.m.

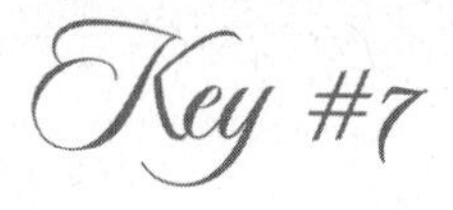

# Key #7

## *Live a Life of Prayer and Purpose*

**Nicki:** After Jordan and I had been married a couple of years, we both came to a similar conclusion at the same time: we would really like to have kids.

I thought I was physically and mentally prepared for the transition to motherhood. On the physical side, I had made a drastic transition in my health since I met Jordan. Now I ate only meats, fruits and vegetables, eggs, cheese, and nuts that were organic. I actually drank water, which is something I had never done with any regularity before. I stopped drinking iced tea because it was unhealthy to flavor it with four teaspoons of sugar. Snacking on an entire bag of Twizzlers was in my past.

One vice remained, however: my love for Starbucks Carmel Macchiatos. I can't remember when I got hooked—it was sometime after the honeymoon—but each time I popped open an eyelid at dawn's first light, it was like this different person got out of bed, put on some clothes and makeup, and drove a mile to the local Starbucks, where she ordered a double tall Carmel Macchiato, organic milk, extra caramel.

The Starbucks *baristas*, like good bartenders, knew my drink of choice as soon as I stepped inside the front door. They even *named* my drink order after me. "Another Nicki, coming right up," a guy with a grin would say from behind the counter. Since a "double tall" meant two shots of espresso, you could say that I was starting the day in a highly caffeinated way.

Jordan was usually fast asleep each morning when I slipped out of bed and made my Starbucks run. On my way home, I would drive slowly through the neighborhood because I had to finish my Carmel Macchiato before I pulled back into the driveway. Disposing of the tall-sized paper cup presented a problem, however, since I didn't want Jordan to find out where I had been. I usually tucked my empty cup under some trash so he wouldn't see it. Sneaking out of the house five mornings a week always gave me a guilty conscience because I *knew* how Jordan felt about sugar-flavored coffee drinks.

I'm sure it wasn't too long before he put two and two together, but he never told me I was dumb or doing something stupid. I remember one time when he found a Starbucks paper cup in the car, and he casually said, "Hey, Honey, you drinking those Starbucks?"—as if it could have been anyone else in our family.

"Yeah, Sweetie, I know they're not good for me, but they taste great."

"Well, they're still not good for you," he said, but he let the matter drop that day.

I'd resist the Starbucks siren call for a few days, but the allure of a sweet coffee drink always brought me back. One time, Jordan caught me sneaking a Starbucks.

"What's in those things?" he asked.

"Well, two shots of espresso, extra caramel sauce, and whipped cream."

"Gosh, how often do you go there anyway?"

"Every day I can, practically. Maybe five days a week."

"Are you addicted?" I'm sure my husband was concerned that he would have to drag me into some twelve-step program.

"No, I'm not addicted. Addicted means you need your coffee or your caffeine. I don't need the caffeine; I just like the way they taste."

The guilt was getting to me, though. Here Jordan was going around the country speaking before audiences about the importance of eating the best foods and drinking the best liquids for the body—and Carmel Macchiatos weren't part of the program. While he was snoozing, his wife was tiptoeing out of the house for her daily java fix.

I could justify my actions, though.

*Look how far you've come.*

*You take all those nutritional supplements, so you're okay.*

*Everything else you eat or drink is what Jordan recommends.*

Meanwhile, we were trying to get pregnant, but after a year, it wasn't happening. I pleaded with the Lord to open up my womb, but my prayers—for whatever reason—went unanswered. At least, that's how I felt.

Then Jordan found research showing that some caffeine-drinking women were having problems getting pregnant. He also felt I was consuming too many carbohydrates, particularly sugar and starches, which meant that I had been raising my insulin levels, a surefire way to produce a hormonal imbalance that could throw my ovulation process off-kilter.

After we looked at all the research, I tried to cut back on my Starbucks runs, but I wasn't perfect. I'd still sneak an occasional Carmel Macchiato when the urge struck me.

Then *two* years passed, and we were still not pregnant. The situation was serious enough for us to schedule an appointment with a fertility specialist to see if there was something physically wrong with either of us. Jordan checked out fine, but as for me, the doctor suspected endometriosis.

Endometriosis, one cause of female infertility, is a condition in which endometrial tissue—the lining inside the uterus—grows *outside* the uterus and attaches to other organs, such as the ovaries and fallopian tubes. My doctor recommended a laparoscopy to remove any ovarian cysts or adhesions in my pelvic cavity and gave me the impression that I would be back on my feet a few days following this outpatient surgery.

By now we were at the two-and-a-half-year point in our quest to bring a child into this world. I was thirty-three years old, not too old to become pregnant, but at an age when it becomes more difficult. Surgery wasn't my preferred route, but if that's what it took, then I was mentally prepared to go under the knife. I chose a date that was a couple of days before Jordan and I planned to go on an Alaskan cruise with Dr. Charles Stanley and his In Touch ministry.

I spoke with a friend who had had the same surgery. When she heard about my plan to leave for the Pacific Northwest two days after the surgery, she shook her head.

"Nicki, you don't want to do that. Trust me, you'll need to rest at least a week. I wouldn't do this surgery if you want to go on the cruise."

I called the doctor's office and said I would reschedule the procedure after my return. Jordan, who wasn't convinced that I had endometriosis, was relieved because he was wary of the surgery.

My husband was busy writing *The Maker's Diet* that summer, and he planned to include a forty-day "health experience" section with a comprehensive meal plan. Before sending the manuscript to the publisher, he wanted to test the plan with three other couples, along with the two of us. That meant I would have to eat "perfect" like Jordan. Nobody eats flawlessly like him, and I told him so.

"It'll be fun," Jordan promised. "We'll meet the other couples for dinner once a week and see how we're all doing. I also think the Maker's Diet can help you get pregnant. Everything else we've tried hasn't worked."

I was listening.

"Tell you what," Jordan said, "if you're not pregnant after three months, then we'll go in for surgery. Promise."

"Okay, I can do that," I said.

I turned on my accountant's mind-set. If the Maker's Diet said no to caffeinated beverages, then no more Starbucks, no more fudging outside the lines. I would not stray one iota from perfection for forty days because I didn't want surgery or fertility drugs, but I wanted a child, so I didn't cheat once during the forty-day health experience.

Then I was late starting my period.

For a couple of years, I had been using an over-the-counter ovulation kit that was supposed to tell me if I ovulated sometime during my cycle. We could never get a positive ovulation reading, which was weird. I was having a normal, twenty-eight-day menstrual cycle, so wasn't I ovulating? While my fertility doctor didn't have a good explanation, Jordan felt all along that it was because of a hormone imbalance related to my diet and lifestyle.

One of my ovulation kits included a pregnancy test. I had never bought a pregnancy test because I had never been late, never thought I could be pregnant. But after a week of waiting, I slipped into the bathroom and performed the test. Presto! Jordan and I were going to be parents.

The news flabbergasted me because we had struggled for so long, prayed so many prayers, and waited thirty months for this good news.

One evening, the discussion turned to when I thought I conceived.

My doctor figured I was six weeks along, so I got out a calendar and counted back. My fingers zeroed in on a certain date in a certain hotel in Springfield, Missouri . . . yup, and I knew exactly when conception occurred.

The truth hit us between the eyes: I had become pregnant on the fortieth day of the Maker's Diet 40-Day Health Experience!

Talk about the Lord answering a prayer in neon lights. For nearly three years, we had beseeched the Lord, asking Him to bless us with a child. At one point, I despaired and said to Jordan, "Well, maybe the Lord doesn't want us to have kids," but Jordan said there were plenty of places in the Bible where a woman was barren for a long time before she became pregnant—sometimes miraculously, sometimes after prayer. Sarah was in her nineties when—miracles of miracles—she bore Isaac. Then Isaac "pleaded with the LORD" (Gen. 25:21 NLT) to give his wife, Rebekah, a child after many years of infertility; she eventually gave birth to twins Jacob and Esau. Jacob's beloved wife, Rachel, was barren for many years until God "answered her prayers by giving her a child" (Gen. 30:22 NLT) with the birth of Joseph.

Prayer is the bridge between heaven and earth. The National Day of Prayer calls prayer the conduit through which the spiritual realm is brought into our everyday lives:

> Prayer is the way our spirits breathe. Just as our lungs require the presence of God and are designed to seek it out, so our spirits require the presence of God and are designed to seek Him out. Without his presence, we are left gasping for meaning and desperately seeking our purpose in life. Prayer is the method God uses to provide not only our daily needs from foods to shelter but also comfort, strength, and guidance.[1]

**Jordan:** Prayer must be foundational to our lives. "Pray without ceasing," says 1 Thessalonians 5:17 (NKJV), which says to me that we need to consciously keep the Lord in our thoughts as we go about our day. One of my favorite books on prayer is *Prayers That Avail Much* by Germaine Copeland. She says that when you confess God's Word in the midst of your prayers to the Almighty, you will experience His amazing power to bring it to fulfillment. Your fervent prayers will avail much, and God will work mightily for you. Her book contains more than 150 prayers covering many different situations: desiring to have a baby, peace in the family, children at school, salvation for the lost, even compatibility in marriage. As an example, here is Mrs. Copeland's prayer for wives:

> Holy Spirit, I ask You to help me understand and support my husband in ways that show my support for Christ. Teach me to function so that I preserve my own personality while responding to his desires. We are one flesh, and I realize that this unity of persons that preserves individuality is a mystery, but that is how it is when we are united to Christ. So I will keep on loving my husband and let the miracle keep happening![2]

**Nicki:** When I became pregnant, Jordan and I were so blown away by the Lord's goodness and mercy, and we genuinely felt we were living in His purpose, although we understand that some women will never be able to get pregnant.

*A Mom's Noble Purpose*
*by Nicki Rubin*

Today, I feel a strong purpose in life: to be a great mom for Joshua as he grows out of infancy and into adulthood. I am part of a continuum that can be traced back through the generations. Joshua's birth was a sacred moment, an awesome experience that brought into sharper focus the miracle of life. When I held my son close to my heart in the birthing room, I knew that God had a wonderful plan for his life, which included my raising him to love the Lord and grow up to become a godly man.

My life had purpose before I met Jordan and before we became parents, but now that I'm a mom, that sense of purpose has sharpened in focus. Every child needs a loving mother, and the timeless love and nurturing that flow from a mother to child will never grow out of fashion. "Who can measure how much a mother's hug means to a crying child?" asked author Beverly LaHaye. "What price tag can we put on a mother who loves and raises a child from infancy to adulthood, while instilling biblical principles that promote not only personal faith but civil responsibility?"[3]

Now, you may be saying, "I'm not sure that God has a great purpose for my life. I'm just a stay-at-home mom; I'm not a doctor or an author. I don't even know that many people, and to tell you the truth, I'm kind of shy."

Some share with me that their husbands tell them that a "man's work" is much more important than what their wives do. The inference is that while the wife is "just" a homemaker, the husband has the major responsibilities in the family. After all, he brings home the bacon. (Well, after reading this book, you need to tell him to stop bringing home the bacon!)

You also need to realize that being a wife and mother is quite possibly the most important and purposeful thing you can do in life. Not only that, whether you work outside the home full-time, part-time, or not at all, you have an opportunity to impact neighbors, friends, or coworkers who are stressed, depressed, broke, sick, and hurting.

Since you have a relationship with the living God, you can make a huge difference in someone else's life. You don't have to be celebrated on the pages of *People* magazine or even speak in front of people publicly. All you have to be is willing and available.

In fact, I bet you've already made a difference in someone else's life, but you may never know the true impact until eternity. Many, many "unknown" people have been used by God to reach millions and millions by adding value to someone's life, one person at a time.

## THE SANDS OF TIME

**Jordan:** Let me give you another example of how your prayers and faithful influence can help others by telling a story that I love to share whenever I speak at a church or a conference:

A little more than a century ago, there was a naturopathic doctor who practiced medicine during the day and gave health seminars in the evenings. Naturopathic doctors use natural methods to treat disease and promote health with the idea that medication should be used as a last resort, instead of the first recommendation.

One evening, among a small crowd of twenty, sat a young man who was suffering from an illness that doctors said was incurable. Instead of giving up, this man attended the naturopathic doctor's health talk and learned how to incorporate natural health principles into his life. After changing his diet and lifestyle, he was not only cured, but he went on to write books and give health lectures.

The young man's name was Norman Walker, who went on to become widely known as the father of colon cleansing and fruit and vegetable juicing. (Norman Walker died in 1985 at more than one hundred years of age.) One afternoon, as he lectured a group of thirty, a young man who was suffering from tuberculosis—an incurable disease at the time—sat in the crowd. Doctors had given up on him, saying there was nothing more they could do. After hearing from Norman Walker about how he could transform his health by following natural, God-given principles, this young man not only overcame tuberculosis, but he went on to share this message of health and hope by giving health seminars and writing books about the benefits of eating healthy, exercising, fasting, and practicing deep breathing. His name was Paul Bragg, and he was considered by many to be the father of the modern "health food" movement before his death at the age of ninety-six—from a surfing accident!

One evening while Paul was teaching, a fifteen-year-old boy sat in the crowd. This young man was suffering from constant headaches, poor digestion, and a low immune system. He was thirty pounds underweight and felt like a weakling. Doctors told him there was nothing that could be done to help him. Inspired by Paul Bragg's message, however, this young man began to eat well and exercise. In a short time, the headaches stopped, his digestion improved, and he gained weight and muscle mass. No one could call him a weakling anymore. He eventually went to chiropractic school and became an avid student of fitness. He gave lectures, authored books, and even hosted one of the first fitness shows on TV.

Today at the age of ninety-two, Jack La Lanne can do more pushups than I can. Not to mention the remarkable feats of strength and endurance he has performed over the years, including towing seventy boats with seventy people from the Queen's Way Bridge in the Long Beach Harbor to the *Queen Mary* for one and a half miles while handcuffed, shackled, and fighting currents.

One night at a Jack La Lanne lecture, a seventeen-year-old boy suffering from a medically incurable upper respiratory condition sat in the audience. Inspired by Jack La Lanne's message that evening, this young man changed his diet and lifestyle and was healed of his condition. This young man went on to dedicate his life to helping people improve their health, giving seminars, and coaching people on how to regain and maintain well-being.

His name was William Keith, whom I doubt you have heard of before. But one day, forty-three years later, William was speaking with a nineteen-year-old teenager who was ill from multiple illnesses, including Crohn's disease, diabetes, arthritis, and countless others, a young man who had visited sixty-nine health professionals who couldn't help him, a young man who had wasted away to just over one hundred pounds and had to be transported in a wheelchair. William Keith told this fellow that if he followed the health principles found in the Bible, then he could be healed from his dreaded diseases.

That nineteen-year-old teen was me, and now that I'm well, I have the privilege of sharing the message of the Great Physician's prescription for women's health with you today, right now. Will *you* be the next link in this chain? Will yours be the next testimony shared with someone who is in need?

Remember, God doesn't call the equipped; He equips the called. Today He could be calling you to get up from where you are, from your painful health challenges, and begin your own health transformation. We serve a great God who forgives all our sins, heals all our diseases, and redeems our lives from destruction, as His Word says in Psalm 103:3–4.

Once your health improves and you've lost weight, have more energy, or have even overcome a serious health challenge, be sure to tell others. Sharing the changes in your life will inspire others and prompt many to ask you how you became so healthy. And you'll answer, "I took a prescription from the Great Physician."

They'll say, "Who's the Great Physician? He sounds important. Is He seeing any patients?"

And then you'll answer, "He sees anyone who comes to Him and asks."

*Are You Ready?*
*by Jordan Rubin*

As you've been reading through this book, have you been following the 49-day health plan that will revolutionize how you—and perhaps your family—will eat and live? If so, who will you be when the forty-nine days are over? Because truth be told, no one stays the same as time passes. You either move forward or decline. Doing the same thing over and over again and expecting a different result, we are told, is the definition of insanity.

I encourage you to take the most important step to your new health and life by giving God the next seven weeks of your life. Allow Him to transform you in body, mind, and spirit. You will be truly amazed at what your life will look like on day 50—the day of jubilee. You will feel different, behave differently, and even look different. You will learn that the secret to being a living sacrifice, as described in Romans 12:1, is a day-to-day discipline of walking on the path that leads to life, which few ever seem to find. Being a living sacrifice is difficult because you can choose to crawl off the altar any time you wish. But God desires your best; God deserves your best.

Some of you will not only transform your life in the next forty-nine days, but many of you may want to lead a small group of women through the 7 Weeks of Wellness program that we've designed. This fantastic small-group curriculum will give you all the tools you need to successfully navigate this life-changing program with your friends and your neighbors.

For more information on leading a 7 Weeks of Wellness group, visit *www.BiblicalHealthInstitute.com.*

For those of you who want to take this message even further, you can enroll in the Biblical Health Coach certification program offered by Biblical Health Institute. This forty-hour online learning program will equip you to take the message of biblical health to your church and your community.

To learn more about becoming a Biblical Health Coach, or to take advantage of the seven free foundational health courses, visit *www.BiblicalHealthInstitute.com.*

*What Women Are Saying*
*by Patricia Lee*

At fifty-two years of age, I'm a young grandma who spends her free time doing dance—ballroom, Latin swing, and praise dance through my church. Around twenty years ago, I had an appendicitis attack and a total hysterectomy, which caused my stomach to bloat out. The weight came on, and as a dancer, I didn't like the way I looked. Then my granddaughter was born three years ago, which was the only positive thing happening in my life because I felt tired all day long. I had fallen into a routine: go to work, come home, sleep some, watch TV or go to church, and then go home and go to bed. I had to quit dancing because I didn't have the energy.

I tried absolutely everything you can imagine—and some things you can't—to turn things around, but nothing worked. Then I read the *Great Physician's Rx for Health and Wellness.* I actually read sections of the book several times to refresh my memory or make sure I understood some of the points Jordan Rubin was trying to get across.

What I liked about the 49-day program was its gradualness. You start out slow and experience small successes, building on each victory until success begets more success. Even when I had a bad day—ate something I knew I shouldn't have—I knew I would succeed at something else on the 49-day wellness plan that day.

I've lost weight, and I've lost inches since I began eating right and incorporating all of the Seven Keys into my life. Instead of waking up three or four times a night, I sleep much more soundly and go through the day having more energy. My seventy-five-year-old mother told me, "Your skin has never looked better," which was encouraging to me. There's joy in my life now.

These days I share the Great Physician's Rx with a lot of people. I've started a 7 Weeks of Wellness small group at my church because I believe in the program so much and because there are people who need to hear about the Bible's principles to unlock their health potential. Oh, and by the way, speaking of classes, I'm teaching praise dance at church as well.

Helping to lead people on a healthy path and into the presence of God is my life purpose, and I could never fulfill that purpose until my health was transformed by God's Word.

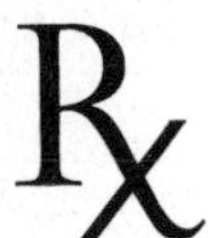

## THE GREAT PHYSICIAN'S Rx FOR WOMEN'S HEALTH: LIVE A LIFE OF PRAYER AND PURPOSE

- *Pray continually, especially when the demands of life and parenting are heavy.*
- *Confess God's promises first thing upon waking and last thing before you retire.*
- *Understand that no matter what stage or season of life you're in, God has a wonderful purpose for your life.*

- *Be an agent of change in your life and the lives of your family. Embark on your own 49-day journey to health and wellness, or consider leading a small group of women through the 7 Weeks of Wellness.*

## THE GREAT PHYSICIAN'S RX FOR WEEK #7

Remember to visit www.BiblicalHealthInstitute.com and click on the GPRx Resource Guide for recommended food, nutritional supplement, advanced hygiene, exercise and body therapy, air and water purification, and skin/body/hair care products.

### DAY 43

*You will notice that some items in the meal plans that follow are italicized. You can find the recipes for these—and over other 250 delicious and healthy recipes—at www.BiblicalHealthInstitute.com.*

***Upon Waking***

*Prayer:* Thank God for His goodness, ask Him to forgive your sins, present your requests to the God who loves you, and read the following Scripture out loud:

> *Bless the LORD, O my soul; and all that is within me, bless His holy name! Bless the LORD, O my soul, and forget not all His benefits: Who forgives all your iniquities, who heals all your diseases, who redeems your life from destruction, who crowns you with lovingkindness and tender mercies, who satisfies your mouth with good things, so that your youth is renewed like the eagle's. (Psalm 103:1–5 NKJV)*

*Purpose:* Ask the Lord to give you an opportunity to add significance to someone's life today. Watch for that opportunity. Ask God to use you this day for His intended purpose.

*Advanced hygiene:* Practice advanced hygiene. See page 277 for guidance.

*Reduce toxins:* Open windows for one hour today. Use natural soap, skin and body care products, facial care products, toothpaste, and hair care products.

*Supplements:* Take one serving of a fiber/green superfood combination containing ground flaxseed, mixed in 12 to 16 ounces of water or raw vegetable juice.

*Body therapy:* Get twenty minutes of direct sunlight.

*Exercise:* Perform functional fitness exercises for fifteen minutes, or spend fifteen minutes on the rebounder. Finish with ten minutes of deep-breathing exercises. During exercise, drink 8 ounces of water.

*Emotional health:* When you face a circumstance that would usually cause you to worry, repeat the following: "Lord, I trust You. I cast my cares upon You, and I believe that You're going to take care of [insert your current situation]." Confess that throughout the day, whenever you think about your circumstance.

*Breakfast*

During breakfast, drink 8 ounces of water.

two eggs (omega-3 or organic, and prepared as desired)

one piece of fruit

one piece of whole-grain sprouted or sourdough toast with butter

hot tea with honey

*Supplements:* Take two whole food multivitamin caplets, one capsule of omega-3 cod-liver oil, and two caplets of a whole food calcium/magnesium blend.

***Between Breakfast and Lunch***

Drink 12 ounces of water.

***Lunch***

During lunch, drink 8 ounces of water.

green salad with two hard-boiled omega-3 eggs, carrots, red onions, cucumbers, and yellow peppers

healthy salad dressing with one tablespoon of extra-virgin olive oil or high-lignan flaxseed oil

one piece of fruit

*Supplements:* Take two whole food multivitamin caplets, one capsule of omega-3 cod-liver oil, and two caplets of a whole food calcium/magnesium blend.

***Between Lunch and Dinner***

Drink 12 ounces of water.

***Dinner***

During dinner, drink 8 ounces of water.

fish of choice

brown rice

grilled asparagus, mushrooms, and onions

green salad with red or yellow peppers, red onions, green or red cabbage, celery, cucumbers, and carrots

healthy salad dressing with olive oil and/or high-lignan flaxseed oil

*Supplements:* Take two whole food multivitamin caplets, one capsule of omega-3 cod-liver oil, and two caplets of a whole food calcium/magnesium blend.

***Snack/Dessert***

apple-cinnamon fiber whole food bar (with beta glucans from soluble oat fiber)

whole-milk yogurt, fruit, and honey

***Before Bed***

*Exercise:* Go for a walk outdoors or participate in a favorite sport or recreational activity. During exercise, drink 8 ounces of water.

*Supplements:* Take one serving of a fiber/green superfood combination containing ground flaxseed, mixed in 12 to 16 ounces of water or raw vegetable juice.

*Body therapy:* Take a warm bath, with eight drops of biblical essential oils added, for fifteen minutes.

*Advanced hygiene:* Practice advanced hygiene.

*Emotional health* (only applicable if there are still people you need to forgive): ask the Lord to bring to your mind someone you need to forgive. Take out a sheet of paper and write the person's name at the top. Try to remember each specific action that person did against you that brought you pain. Write down the following: "I forgive [insert person's name] for [insert the action he or she did against you]." After you fill up the paper, tear it up or burn it, and ask God to give you the strength to truly forgive that person.

*Purpose:* Ask yourself this question: "Did I live a life of purpose today?" What did you do to add value to someone else's life today? Commit to living a day of purpose tomorrow.

*Prayer:* Thank God for this day, asking Him to give you a restoring night's rest and a fresh start tomorrow. Thank Him for His steadfast love that never ceases, and His mercies, which are new every morning. Read the following Scripture out loud:

> *But those who wait on the LORD shall renew their strength; they shall mount up with wings like eagles, they shall run and not be weary, they shall walk and not faint. (Isa. 40:31 NKJV)*

*Sleep:* Go to bed by 10:30 p.m.

## DAY 44

*You will notice that some items in the meal plans that follow are italicized. You can find the recipes for these—and over other 250 delicious and healthy recipes—at www.BiblicalHealthInstitute.com.*

***Upon Waking***

*Prayer:* Thank God for His goodness, ask Him to forgive your sins, present your requests to the God who loves you, and read the following Scripture out loud:

> *Fear not, for I have redeemed you; I have called you by your name; you are mine. When you pass through the waters, I will be with you; and through the rivers, they shall not overflow you. When you walk through the fire, you shall not be burned, nor shall the flame scorch you. (Isa. 43:1b–2 NKJV)*

*Purpose:* Ask the Lord to give you an opportunity to add significance to someone's life today. Watch for that opportunity. Ask God to use you this day for His intended purpose.

*Advanced hygiene:* Practice advanced hygiene. See page 277 for guidance.

*Reduce toxins:* Open windows for one hour today. Use natural soap, skin and body care products, facial care products, toothpaste, and hair care products.

*Supplements:* Take one serving of a fiber/green superfood combination containing ground flaxseed, mixed in 12 to 16 ounces of water or raw vegetable juice.

*Exercise:* Perform functional fitness exercises for fifteen minutes, or spend fifteen minutes on the rebounder. Finish with ten minutes of deep-breathing exercises. During exercise, drink 8 ounces of water.

*Body therapy:* Take a hot-and-cold shower.

*Emotional health:* When you face a circumstance that would usually cause you to worry, repeat the following: "Lord, I trust You. I cast my cares upon You, and I believe that You're going to take care of [insert your current situation]." Confess that throughout the day, whenever you think about your circumstance.

***Breakfast***

During breakfast, drink 8 ounces of water.

For a healthy smoothie, mix the following in a blender:

8 ounces plain whole milk, yogurt, or kefir

1 tablespoon honey

1/2 cup fresh or frozen fruit (bananas, peaches, berries, pineapple, etc.)

1 teaspoon high-lignan flaxseed oil

1 serving of protein powder (optional)

hot tea with honey

*Supplements:* Take two whole food multivitamin caplets, one capsule of omega-3 cod-liver oil, and two caplets of a whole food calcium/magnesium blend.

***Between Breakfast and Lunch***

Drink 12 ounces of water.

***Lunch***

During lunch, drink 8 ounces of water.

low-mercury, high omega-3 tuna on sprouted or yeast-free whole-grain bread with lettuce, tomato, and sprouts

one piece of fruit

*Supplements:* Take two whole food multivitamin caplets, one capsule of omega-3 cod-liver oil, and two caplets of a whole food calcium/magnesium blend.

***Between Lunch and Dinner***

Drink 12 ounces of water.

***Dinner***

During dinner, drink 8 ounces of water.

chicken of choice

steamed broccoli

green salad with red or yellow peppers, red onions, green or red cabbage, celery, cucumbers, and carrots

healthy salad dressing with olive oil and/or high-lignan flaxseed oil

*Simple Lentils*

*Supplements:* Take two whole food multivitamin caplets, one capsule of omega-3 cod-liver oil, and two caplets of a whole food calcium/magnesium blend.

***Snack/Dessert***

whole food meal replacement powder (with beta-glucans from soluble oat fiber) mixed in 12 ounces of water

one piece of fruit and one ounce of cheese

***Before Bed***

*Exercise:* Go for a walk outdoors or participate in a favorite sport or recreational activity. During exercise, drink 8 ounces of water.

*Supplements:* Take one serving of a fiber/green superfood combination containing ground flaxseed, mixed in 12 to 16 ounces of water or raw vegetable juice.

*Advanced hygiene:* Practice advanced hygiene.

*Emotional health* (only applicable if there are still people you need to forgive): Ask the Lord to bring to your mind someone you need to forgive. Take out a sheet of paper and write the person's name at the top. Try to remember each specific action that person did against you that brought you pain. Write down the following: "I forgive [insert person's name] for [insert the action he or she did against you]." After you fill up the paper, tear it up or burn it, and ask God to give you the strength to truly forgive that person.

*Purpose:* Ask yourself this question: "Did I live a life of purpose today?" What did you do to add value to someone else's life today? Commit to living a day of purpose tomorrow.

*Prayer:* Thank God for this day, asking Him to give you a restoring night's rest and a fresh start tomorrow. Thank Him for His steadfast love that never ceases, and His mercies, which are new every morning. Read the following Scripture out loud:

> *Give unto the LORD the glory due to His name; worship the LORD in the beauty of holiness. The voice of the LORD is over the waters; the God of glory thunders; the LORD is over many waters. The voice of the LORD is powerful; the voice of the LORD is full of majesty. (Ps. 29:2–4 NKJV)*

*Body therapy:* Spend ten minutes listening to soothing music before you retire.

*Sleep:* Go to bed by 10:30 p.m.

## DAY 45

*You will notice that some items in the meal plans that follow are italicized. You can find the recipes for these—and over other 250 delicious and healthy recipes—at www.BiblicalHealthInstitute.com.*

***Upon Waking***

*Prayer:* Thank God for His goodness, ask Him to forgive your sins, present your requests to the God who loves you, and read the following Scripture out loud:

*That He would grant you, according to the riches of His glory, to be strengthened with might through His Spirit in the inner man, that Christ may dwell in your hearts through faith; that you, being rooted and grounded in love, may be able to comprehend with all the saints what is the width and length and depth and height—to know the love of Christ which passes knowledge; that you may be filled with all the fullness of God. Now to Him who is able to do exceedingly abundantly above all that we ask or think, according to the power that works in us, to Him be glory in the church by Christ Jesus to all generations, forever and ever. Amen. (Eph. 3:16–21 NKJV)*

*Purpose:* Ask the Lord to give you an opportunity to add significance to someone's life today. Watch for that opportunity. Ask God to use you this day for His intended purpose.

*Advanced hygiene:* Practice advanced hygiene. See page 277 for guidance.

*Reduce toxins:* Open windows for one hour today. Use natural soap, skin and body care products, facial care products, toothpaste, and hair care products.

*Supplements:* Take one serving of a fiber/green superfood combination containing ground flaxseed, mixed in 12 to 16 ounces of water or raw vegetable juice.

*Exercise:* Perform functional fitness exercises for fifteen minutes, or spend fifteen minutes on the rebounder. Finish with ten minutes of deep-breathing exercises. During exercise, drink 8 ounces of water.

*Body therapy:* Get twenty minutes of direct sunlight.

*Emotional health:* When you face a circumstance that would usually cause you to worry, repeat the following: "Lord, I trust You. I cast my cares upon You, and I believe that You're going to take care of [insert your current situation]." Confess that throughout the day, whenever you think about your circumstance.

***Breakfast***

During breakfast, drink 8 ounces of water.

sprouted dry cereal with yogurt, goat's milk, or almond milk.

banana

hot tea with honey

*Supplements:* Take two whole food multivitamin caplets, one capsule of omega-3 cod-liver oil, and two caplets of a whole food calcium/magnesium blend.

***Between Breakfast and Lunch***

Drink 12 ounces of water.

***Lunch***

During lunch, drink 8 ounces of water.

green salad with 3 ounces of tuna (low-mercury, high omega-3) and carrots, red onions, cucumbers, and yellow peppers

healthy salad dressing with one tablespoon of extra-virgin olive oil or high-lignan flaxseed oil

one piece of fruit

*Supplements:* Take two whole food multivitamin caplets, one capsule of omega-3 cod-liver oil, and two caplets of a whole food calcium/magnesium blend.

***Between Lunch and Dinner***

Drink 12 ounces of water.

***Dinner***

During dinner, drink 8 ounces of water.

fish of choice

brown rice

miso soup

green salad with red or yellow peppers, red onions, green or red cabbage, celery, cucumbers, and carrots

healthy salad dressing with olive oil and/or high-lignan flaxseed oil

*Supplements:* Take two whole food multivitamin caplets, one capsule of omega-3 cod-liver oil, and two caplets of a whole food calcium/magnesium blend.

***Snack/Dessert***

berry antioxidant whole food bar (with beta-glucans from soluble oat fiber)

apple with almond or sesame butter (tahini)

***Before Bed***

*Exercise:* Go for a walk outdoors or participate in a favorite sport or recreational activity. During exercise, drink 8 ounces of water.

*Supplements:* Take one serving of a fiber/green superfood combination containing ground flaxseed, mixed in 12 to 16 ounces of water or raw vegetable juice.

*Advanced hygiene:* Practice advanced hygiene.

*Emotional health* (only applicable if there are still people you need to forgive): Ask the Lord to bring to your mind someone you need to forgive. Take out a sheet of paper and write the person's name at the top. Try to remember each specific action that person did against you that brought you pain. Write down the following: "I forgive [insert person's name] for [insert the action he or she did against you]." After you fill up the paper, tear it up or burn it, and ask God to give you the strength to truly forgive that person.

*Body therapy:* Take a warm bath, with eight drops of biblical essential oils added, for fifteen minutes.

*Purpose:* Ask yourself this question: "Did I live a life of purpose today?" What did you do to add value to someone else's life today? Commit to living a day of purpose tomorrow.

*Prayer:* Thank God for this day, asking Him to give you a restoring night's rest and a fresh start tomorrow. Thank Him for His steadfast love that never ceases, and His mercies, which are new every morning. Read the following Scripture out loud:

> *I am the vine, you are the branches. He who abides in Me, and I in him, bears much fruit; for without Me you can do nothing . . . If you abide in Me, and My words abide in you, you will ask what you desire, and it shall be done for you. (John 15:5, 7 NKJV)*

*Sleep:* Go to bed by 10:30 p.m.

## DAY 46

*You will notice that some items in the meal plans that follow are italicized. You can find the recipes for these—and over other 250 delicious and healthy recipes—at www.BiblicalHealthInstitute.com.*

*Upon Waking*

*Prayer:* Thank God for His goodness, ask Him to forgive your sins, present your requests to the God who loves you, and read the following Scripture out loud:

> *Who can find a virtuous wife? For her worth is far above rubies. The heart of her husband safely trusts her; so he will have no lack of gain. She does him good and not evil all the days of her life. She seeks wool and flax, and willingly works with her hands. She is like the merchant ships, she brings her food from afar. She also rises while it is yet night, and provides food for her household, and a portion for her maidservants. She considers a field and buys it; from her profits she plants a vineyard. She girds herself with strength, and strengthens her arms. She perceives that her merchandise is good, and her lamp does not go out by night. She stretches out her hands to the distaff, and her hand holds the spindle. She extends her hand to the poor, yes, she reaches out her hands to the needy. She is not afraid of snow for her household, for all her household is clothed with scarlet. She makes tapestry for herself; Her clothing is fine linen and purple. Her husband is known in the gates, when he sits among the elders of the land. She makes linen garments and sells them, and supplies sashes for the merchants. Strength and honor are her clothing; she shall rejoice in time to come. She opens her mouth with wisdom, and on her tongue is the law of kindness. She watches over the ways of her household, and does not eat the bread of idleness. Her children rise up and call her blessed; her husband also, and he praises her: "Many daughters have done well, but you excel them all." Charm is deceitful and beauty is passing, but a woman who fears the LORD, she shall be praised. Give her of the fruit of her hands, and let her own works praise her in the gates. (Prov. 31:10–31 NKJV)*

*Purpose:* Ask the Lord to give you an opportunity to add significance to someone's life today. Watch for that opportunity. Ask God to use you this day for His intended purpose.

*Advanced hygiene:* Practice advanced hygiene. See page 277 for guidance.

*Reduce toxins:* Open windows for one hour today. Use natural soap, skin and body care products, facial care products, toothpaste, and hair care products.

*Supplements:* Take one serving of a fiber/green superfood combination containing ground flaxseed, mixed in 12 to 16 ounces of water or raw vegetable juice.

*Exercise:* Perform functional fitness exercises for fifteen minutes, or spend fifteen minutes on the rebounder. Finish with ten minutes of deep-breathing exercises. During exercise, drink 8 ounces of water.

*Body therapy:* Take a hot-and-cold shower.

*Emotional health:* When you face a circumstance that would usually cause you to worry, repeat the following: "Lord, I trust You. I cast my cares upon You, and I believe that You're going to take care of [insert your current situation]." Confess that throughout the day, whenever you think about your circumstance.

***Breakfast***

During breakfast, drink 8 ounces of water.

For a healthy smoothie, mix the following in a blender:

8 ounces plain whole milk, yogurt, or kefir

1 tablespoon honey

1/2 cup fresh or frozen fruit (bananas, peaches, berries, pineapple, etc.)

1 teaspoon high-lignan flaxseed oil

1 serving of protein powder (optional)

*Supplements:* Take two whole food multivitamin caplets, one capsule of omega-3 cod-liver oil, and two caplets of a whole food calcium/magnesium blend.

***Between Breakfast and Lunch***

Drink 12 ounces of water.

***Lunch***

During lunch, drink 8 ounces of water

turkey on sprouted or yeast-free whole-grain bread with lettuce, tomato, and sprouts

one piece of fruit

*Supplements:* Take two whole food multivitamin caplets, one capsule of omega-3 cod-liver oil, and two caplets of a whole food calcium/magnesium blend.

*Between Lunch and Dinner*

Drink 12 ounces of water.

*Dinner*

During dinner, drink 8 ounces of water.

wild salmon

steamed broccoli

baked sweet potato

green salad with red or yellow peppers, red onions, green or red cabbage, celery, cucumbers, and carrots

healthy salad dressing with olive oil and/or high-lignan flaxseed oil

*Supplements:* Take two whole food multivitamin caplets, one capsule of omega-3 cod-liver oil, and two caplets of a whole food calcium/magnesium blend.

*Snack/Dessert*

whole food meal replacement powder (with beta-glucans from soluble oat fiber) mixed in 12 ounces of water

raw veggies and hummus, salsa, or guacamole

*Before Bed*

*Exercise:* Go for a walk outdoors or participate in a favorite sport or recreational activity. During exercise, drink 8 ounces of water.

*Supplements:* Take one serving of a fiber/green superfood combination containing ground flaxseed, mixed in 12 to 16 ounces of water or raw vegetable juice.

*Advanced hygiene:* Practice advanced hygiene.

*Emotional health* (only applicable if there are still people you need to forgive): Ask the Lord to bring to your mind someone you need to forgive. Take out a sheet of paper and write the person's name at the top. Try to remember each specific action that person did against you that brought you pain. Write down the following: "I forgive [insert person's name] for [insert the action he or she did against you]." After you fill up the paper, tear it up or burn it, and ask God to give you the strength to truly forgive that person.

*Purpose:* Ask yourself, "Did I live a life of purpose today?" What did you do to add value to someone else's life today? Commit to living a day of purpose tomorrow.

*Prayer:* Thank God for this day, asking Him to give you a restoring night's rest and a fresh start tomorrow. Thank Him for His steadfast love that never ceases, and His mercies, which are new every morning. Read the following Scripture out loud:

> *O LORD my God, I cried out to You, and You healed me . . . Sing praise to the LORD, you saints of His, and give thanks at the remembrance of His holy name. For His anger is but for a moment, His favor is for life; weeping may endure for a night, but joy comes in the morning . . . LORD, by Your favor You have made my mountain stand strong; You hid Your face, and I was troubled . . . You have turned for me my mourning into dancing; You have put off my sackcloth and clothed me with gladness, to the end that my glory may sing praise to You and not be silent. O LORD my God, I will give thanks to You forever. (Ps. 30:2, 4–5, 7, 11–12 NKJV)*

*Body therapy:* Spend ten minutes listening to soothing music before you retire.

*Sleep:* Go to bed by 10:30 p.m.

## DAY 47 (PARTIAL-FAST DAY)

*You will notice that some items in the meal plans that follow are italicized. You can find the recipes for these—and over other 250 delicious and healthy recipes—at www.BiblicalHealthInstitute.com.*

***Upon Waking***

*Prayer:* Thank God for His goodness, ask Him to forgive your sins, present your requests to the God who loves you, and read the following Scripture out loud:

> *Is this not the fast that I have chosen: to loose the bonds of wickedness, to undo the heavy burdens, to let the oppressed go free, and that you break every yoke? . . . Then your light shall break forth like the morning, your healing shall spring forth speedily, and your righteousness shall go before you; the glory of the LORD shall be your*

*rear guard. Then you shall call, and the Lord will answer; you shall cry, and He will say, "Here I am." (Isa. 58:6, 8–9 NKJV)*

*Purpose:* Ask the Lord to give you an opportunity to add significance to someone's life today. Watch for that opportunity. Ask God to use you this day for His intended purpose.

*Advanced hygiene:* Practice advanced hygiene. See page 277 for guidance.

*Reduce toxins:* Open windows for one hour today. Use natural soap, skin and body care products, facial care products, toothpaste, and hair care products.

*Supplements:* Take one serving of a fiber/green superfood combination containing ground flaxseed, mixed in 12 to 16 ounces of water or raw vegetable juice.

*Exercise:* Perform functional fitness exercises for fifteen minutes, or spend fifteen minutes on the rebounder. Finish with ten minutes of deep-breathing exercises. During exercise, drink 8 ounces of water.

*Body therapy:* Get twenty minutes of direct sunlight.

*Emotional health:* When you face a circumstance that would usually cause you to worry, repeat the following: "Lord, I trust You. I cast my cares upon You, and I believe that You're going to take care of [insert your current situation]." Confess that throughout the day, whenever you think about your circumstance.

***Breakfast***

none (partial-fast day)

Drink 12 ounces of water.

*Supplements:* Take two whole food multivitamin caplets, one capsule of omega-3 cod-liver oil, and two caplets of a whole food calcium/magnesium blend.

***Between Breakfast and Lunch***

Drink 12 ounces of water.

***Lunch***

none (partial-fast day)

Drink 12 ounces of water.

***Between Lunch and Dinner***

Drink 12 ounces of water.

***Dinner***

During dinner, drink 8 ounces of water.

*Chicken Soup*

fermented vegetables

*Oriental Salmon Salad*

*Supplements:* Take two whole food multivitamin caplets, one capsule of omega-3 cod-liver oil, and two caplets of a whole food calcium/magnesium blend.

***Snack/Dessert***

none (partial-fast day)

Drink 12 ounces of water.

***Before Bed***

Drink 8–12 ounces of water or hot tea with honey.

*Exercise:* Go for a walk outdoors or participate in a favorite sport or recreational activity. During exercise, drink 8 ounces of water.

*Supplements:* Take one serving of a fiber/green superfood combination containing ground flaxseed, mixed in 12 to 16 ounces of water or raw vegetable juice.

*Advanced hygiene:* Practice advanced hygiene.

*Emotional health* (only applicable if there are still people you need to forgive): Ask the Lord to bring to your mind someone you need to forgive. Take out a sheet of paper and write the person's name at the top. Try to remember each specific action that person did against you that brought you pain. Write down the following: "I forgive [insert person's name] for [insert the action he or she did against you]." After you fill up the paper, tear it up or burn it, and ask God to give you the strength to truly forgive that person.

*Body therapy:* Take a warm bath, with eight drops of biblical essential oils added, for fifteen minutes.

*Purpose:* Ask yourself, "Did I live a life of purpose today?" What did you do to add value to someone else's life today? Commit to living a day of purpose tomorrow.

*Prayer:* Thank God for this day, asking Him to give you a restoring night's rest and a fresh start tomorrow. Thank Him for His steadfast love that never ceases, and His mercies, which are new every morning. Read this morning's Scripture out loud again:

> *Is this not the fast that I have chosen: to loose the bonds of wickedness, to undo the heavy burdens, to let the oppressed go free, and that you break every yoke? . . . Then your light shall break forth like the morning, your healing shall spring forth speedily, and your righteousness shall go before you; the glory of the LORD shall be your rear guard. Then you shall call, and the LORD will answer; you shall cry, and He will say, "Here I am." (Isa. 58:6, 8–9 NKJV)*

*Sleep:* Go to bed by 10:30 p.m.

## DAY 48 (DAY OF REST)

*You will notice that some items in the meal plans that follow are italicized. You can find the recipes for these—and over other 250 delicious and healthy recipes—at www.BiblicalHealthInstitute.com.*

***Upon Waking***

*Prayer:* Thank God for His goodness, ask Him to forgive your sins, present your requests to the God who loves you, and read the following Scripture out loud:

> *I will bless the LORD at all times; His praise shall continually be in my mouth. My soul shall make its boast in the LORD; the humble shall hear of it and be glad. Oh, magnify the LORD with me, and let us exalt His name together. I sought the LORD, and He heard me, and delivered me from all my fears. They looked to Him and were radiant, and their faces were not ashamed. This poor man cried out, and the LORD heard him, and saved him out of all his troubles. The angel of the LORD encamps all around those who fear Him, and delivers them. Oh, taste and see that the LORD is good; blessed is the man who trusts in Him! Oh, fear the LORD, you His saints! There is no want to those who fear Him (Ps. 34:1–9 NKJV).*

*Purpose:* Ask the Lord to give you an opportunity to add significance to someone's life today. Watch for that opportunity. Ask God to use you this day for His intended purpose.

*Advanced hygiene:* Practice advanced hygiene. See page 277 for guidance.

*Reduce toxins:* Open windows for one hour today. Use natural soap, skin and body care products, facial care products, toothpaste, and hair care products.

*Supplements:* Take one serving of a fiber/green superfood combination containing ground flaxseed, mixed in 12 to 16 ounces of water or raw vegetable juice.

*Exercise:* None

*Body therapies:* None

*Emotional health:* When you face a circumstance that would usually cause you to worry, repeat the following: "Lord, I trust You. I cast my cares upon You, and I believe that You're going to take care of [insert your current situation]." Confess that throughout the day, whenever you think about your circumstance.

***Breakfast***

During breakfast, drink 8 ounces of water.

sprouted or raw dry cereal

4 ounces of whole-milk yogurt or goat's milk

raw honey

fresh fruit

hot tea with honey

*Supplements:* Take two whole food multivitamin caplets, one capsule of omega-3 cod-liver oil, and two caplets of a whole food calcium/magnesium blend.

***Between Breakfast and Lunch***

Drink 12 ounces of water.

***Lunch***

During lunch, drink 8 ounces of water.

green salad with 3 ounces of salmon and carrots, red onions, cucumbers, and yellow peppers

healthy salad dressing with one tablespoon of extra-virgin olive oil or high-lignan flaxseed oil

one piece of fruit

*Supplements:* Take two whole food multivitamin caplets, one capsule of omega-3 cod-liver oil, and two caplets of a whole food calcium/magnesium blend.

***Between Lunch and Dinner***

Drink 12 ounces of water.

***Dinner***

During dinner, drink 8 ounces of water.

*Chicken Soup*

chicken of choice

quinoa

*Sautéed Veggies*

green salad with red or yellow peppers, red onions, green or red cabbage, celery, cucumbers, and carrots

healthy salad dressing with olive oil and/or high-lignan flaxseed oil

*Supplements:* Take two whole food multivitamin caplets, one capsule of omega-3 cod-liver oil, and two caplets of a whole food calcium/magnesium blend.

***Snack/Dessert***

green superfood whole food bar (with beta-glucans from soluble oat fiber)

raw nuts, seeds, and dried fruit

***Before Bed***

*Exercise:* Go for a walk outdoors or participate in a favorite sport or recreational activity. During exercise, drink 8 ounces of water.

*Supplements:* Take one serving of a fiber/green superfood combination containing ground flaxseed, mixed in 12 to 16 ounces of water or raw vegetable juice.

*Advanced hygiene:* Practice advanced hygiene.

*Emotional health* (only applicable if there are still people you need to forgive): Ask the Lord to bring to your mind someone you need to forgive. Take out a sheet of paper and write the person's name at the top. Try to remember each specific action that person did against you that brought you pain. Write down the following: "I forgive [insert person's name] for [insert the action he or she did against you]." After you fill up the paper, tear it up or burn it, and ask God to give you the strength to truly forgive that person.

*Purpose:* Ask yourself, "Did I live a life of purpose today?" What did you do to add value to someone else's life today? Commit to living a day of purpose tomorrow.

*Prayer:* Thank God for this day, asking Him to give you a restoring night's rest and a fresh start tomorrow. Thank Him for His steadfast love that never ceases, and His mercies, which are new every morning. Read the following Scripture out loud:

> *My son, do not forget my law, but let your heart keep my commands; for length of days and long life and peace they will add to you. Let not mercy and truth forsake you; bind them around your neck, write them on the tablet of your heart, and so find favor and high esteem in the sight of God and man. Trust in the LORD with all your heart, and lean not on your own understanding; in all your ways acknowledge Him, and He shall direct your paths. Do not be wise in your own eyes; fear the LORD and depart from evil. It will be health to your flesh, and strength to your bones. Honor the LORD with your possessions, and with the firstfruits of all your increase; so your barns will be filled with plenty, and your vats will overflow with new wine.* (Prov. 3:1–10 NKJV)

*Body therapy:* Spend ten minutes listening to soothing music before you retire.

*Sleep:* Go to bed by 10:30 p.m.

## Day 49

*You will notice that some items in the meal plans that follow are italicized. You can find the recipes for these—and over other 250 delicious and healthy recipes—at www.BiblicalHealthInstitute.com.*

***Upon Waking***

*Prayer:* Thank God for His goodness, ask Him to forgive your sins, present your requests to the God who loves you, and read the following Scripture out loud:

> *Create in me a clean heart, O God, and renew a steadfast spirit within me. Do not cast me away from Your presence, and do not take Your Holy Spirit from me. Restore to me the joy of Your salvation, and uphold me by Your generous Spirit.* (Ps. 51:10–12 NKJV)

*Purpose:* Ask the Lord to give you an opportunity to add significance to someone's life today. Watch for that opportunity. Ask God to use you this day for His intended purpose.

*Advanced hygiene:* Practice advanced hygiene. See page 277 for guidance.

*Reduce toxins:* Open windows for one hour today. Use natural soap, skin and body care products, facial care products, toothpaste, and hair care products.

*Supplements:* Take one serving of a fiber/green superfood combination containing ground flaxseed, mixed in 12 to 16 ounces of water or raw vegetable juice.

*Exercise:* Perform functional fitness exercises for fifteen minutes, or spend fifteen minutes on the rebounder. Finish with ten minutes of deep-breathing exercises. During exercise, drink 8 ounces of water.

*Body therapy:* Get twenty minutes of direct sunlight.

*Emotional health:* When you face a circumstance that would usually cause you to worry, repeat the following: "Lord, I trust You. I cast my cares upon You, and I believe that You're going to take care of [insert your current situation]." Confess that throughout the day, whenever you think about your circumstance.

***Breakfast***

During breakfast, drink 8 ounces of water.

two-egg omelet with avocado, cheese, tomato, onion, and pepper

*Sautéed Veggies*

hot tea and honey

*Supplements:* Take two whole food multivitamin caplets, one capsule of omega-3 cod-liver oil, and two caplets of a whole food calcium/magnesium blend.

***Between Breakfast and Lunch***

Drink 12 ounces of water.

***Lunch***

During lunch, drink 8 ounces of water.

almond butter and honey or pure fruit jam on sprouted or yeast-free whole-grain bread with lettuce, tomato, and sprouts

one piece of fruit

*Supplements:* Take two whole food multivitamin caplets, one capsule of omega-3 cod-liver oil, and two caplets of a whole food calcium/magnesium blend.

***Between Lunch and Dinner***

Drink 12 ounces of water.

***Dinner***

During dinner, drink 8 ounces of water.

red meat of choice

*Garlicky Green Beans*

green salad with red or yellow peppers, red onions, green or red cabbage, celery, cucumbers, and carrots

healthy salad dressing with olive oil and/or high-lignan flaxseed oil

*Supplements:* Take two whole food multivitamin caplets, one capsule of omega-3 cod-liver oil, and two caplets of a whole food calcium/magnesium blend.

***Snack/Dessert***

whole food meal replacement powder (with beta-glucans from soluble oat fiber) mixed in 12 ounces of water

*Raw Fruit Pie* with a date and nut crust

***Before Bed***

*Exercise:* Go for a walk outdoors or participate in a favorite sport or recreational activity. During exercise, drink 8 ounces of water.

*Supplements:* Take one serving of a fiber/green superfood combination containing ground flaxseed, mixed in 12 to 16 ounces of water or raw vegetable juice.

*Advanced hygiene:* Practice advanced hygiene.

*Emotional health* (only applicable if there are still people you need to forgive): Ask the Lord to bring to your mind someone you need to forgive. Take out a sheet of paper and write the person's name at the top. Try to remember each specific action that person did against you that brought you pain. Write down the following: "I forgive [insert person's name] for [insert the action he or she did against you]." After you fill up the paper, tear it up or burn it, and ask God to give you the strength to truly forgive that person.

*Body therapy:* Take a warm bath, with eight drops of biblical essential oils added, for fifteen minutes.

*Purpose:* Ask yourself, "Did I live a life of purpose today?" What did you do to add value to someone else's life today? Commit to living a day of purpose tomorrow.

*Prayer:* Thank God for this day, asking Him to give you a restoring night's rest and a fresh start tomorrow. Thank Him for His steadfast love that never ceases, and His mercies, which are new every morning. Read the following Scripture out loud:

> *And He said to me, "My grace is sufficient for you, for My strength is made perfect in weakness." Therefore most gladly I will rather boast in my infirmities, that the power of Christ may rest upon me. Therefore I take pleasure in infirmities, in reproaches, in needs, in persecutions, in distresses, for Christ's sake. For when I am weak, then I am strong."* (2 Cor. 12:9–10 NKJV)

*Sleep:* Go to bed by 10:30 p.m.

## DAY 50 (JUBILEE DAY)

*Proclaim liberty throughout all the land to all its inhabitants. It shall be a Jubilee for you.*
—Leviticus 25:10 NKJV

If you have been faithful to the Great Physician's Rx for the last forty-nine days, then I offer you heartfelt congratulations. This is the day to celebrate your success and renewed physical, mental, emotional, and spiritual health. Treat yourself to any foods you want, except for the Dirty Dozen, of course.

If you still have a little farther to go, however—some pounds to lose, high blood pressure to deal with, some achy joints or unresolved digestive complaints—I encourage you to stay on the Great Physician's prescription for health and wellness.

If you're happy with your newfound level of health and want to continue your lifetime of wellness, I encourage you to log onto www.BiblicalHealthInstitute.com and embark on the Lifetime of Wellness plan. This plan incorporates all of the principles of the *Great Physician's Rx for Women's Health* with the special three-cheats-a-week bonus meals. The Lifetime of Wellness plan is simply the most doable and effective health plan for you and your family.

Allow me to pray over you the priestly blessing from Numbers 6:24–26 (NKJV):

*The LORD bless you and keep you*
*the LORD make His face shine upon you,*
*and be gracious to you*
*the LORD lift up His countenance upon you,*
*and give you peace.*
*In the name of the Lord Jesus, our Messiah,*
*Amen.*

# A Refresher on Practicing Advanced Hygiene

For hands and nails, jab fingers into semisoft soap four or five times, and lather hands for fifteen seconds, rubbing soap over cuticles and rinsing under water as warm as you can stand. Use another scoop of semisoft soap to wash your face.

Next, fill basin or sink with water as warm as you can stand, and add one-to-three tablespoons of table salt and one-to-three eyedroppers of iodine-based mineral solution. Swirl water. Dunk face into water and open eyes, blinking repeatedly under water. Keep eyes open under water for three seconds.

After cleaning your eyes, put your face back in the water, and close your mouth while blowing bubbles out of your nose. Come up from the water, and immerse your nose in the water once again, gently taking water into your nostrils and expelling bubbles. Come up from the water, and blow your nose into facial tissue.

To cleanse the ears, use hydrogen peroxide and mineral-based ear drops, putting two or three drops into each ear and letting stand for sixty seconds. Tilt your head to expel the drops. For the teeth, apply two or three drops of essential oil–based tooth drops to the toothbrush. This can be used to brush your teeth or can be added to existing toothpaste. After brushing your teeth, brush your tongue for fifteen seconds.

You can visit www.BiblicalHealthInstitute.com to learn more about recommended advanced hygiene products.

# Appendix
## Real-Life Transformations

To facilitate my mission to transform the health of God's people one life at a time, I minister nearly every weekend to churches by sharing the message of the Great Physician's Rx. One great church I had the privilege to minister to was Calvary Temple Worship Center in Modesto, California, pastored by Glen Berteau. The pastoral team and congregation responded so well to the message that Calvary Temple hosted a 7 Weeks of Wellness challenge to take the health of their church to the next level. More than 360 men and women participated.

Each week, participants listened as Kelli Williams, the health ministries pastor *and* a registered nurse, facilitated each of the Seven Keys utilizing our 7 Weeks of Wellness church curriculum. After hearing excellent testimonies about how lives were transformed, I asked some of the women to share how filling the prescription from the Great Physician had changed their lives.

*Bring the 7 Weeks of Wellness to Your Hometown!*

You can transform the health of your friends and neighbors by asking your church to facilitate a 7 Weeks of Wellness program, or you can lead a small group on your own. For more information on the 7 Weeks of Wellness small-group resources, visit www.BiblicalHealthInstitute.com.

### Christy Utterback

I'm a single mother who often has to work long hours, so eating on the run became a habit for me. Hearing Jordan speak on what God's Word says about health and the foods we should eat convicted me to change my dietary habits. While I'm blessed that I haven't had any major illnesses, I was left wondering why I had been jeopardizing my health by consuming food that is convenient and fast.

I started by cleaning out my cupboards and throwing away everything in the "Dirty Dozen" category. I used to dread grocery shopping, but after starting to shop at a health food store, I actually left the market feeling good about the healthy choices I made for my daughter, Alexis, and myself. Since we've started eating foods that God created, she has stopped taking her allergy and asthma medications.

I've also been practicing advanced hygiene each morning and evening. Adding it to my daily routine has helped me take the time to focus more on prevention, which Jordan says is the only 100-percent cure. Surprisingly, even my five-year-old Alexis loves "sink snorkeling." She opens her eyes and sucks in the water through her nose. Last summer she wouldn't even go underwater in the pool, and now she's dunking her head every night!

We just finished remodeling our home, and we incorporated an air filtration system and water purifier so we can start off in the right direction. Next year, I plan to change my pool to a natural salt cleaning system instead of using chlorine.

I've noticed such a difference in my life after making these changes. My energy level has skyrocketed, and my hunger for the Lord has increased dramatically. I find myself mentally and physically capable to handle more for ministry. I lost eight pounds during the 7 Weeks of Wellness and didn't find myself wanting to snack in the middle of the day.

One time, though, I went out for a greasy lunch with a friend and had to go home from work early because I had a terrible stomachache. I will never go back to eating detestable and unclean foods, because I want to keep my body, His temple, clean and pure.

### CAROL WOOTEN

Last year I got very sick with a staph infection in my knee. I also was battling high blood pressure and very high blood sugar. Following Jordan's 7 Weeks of Wellness program lowered my blood sugar level to normal. I'm off blood pressure meds, and now I have to take insulin for my diabetes just once a day—if that—after previously having to take four shots a day. My cholesterol is now 91 points lower, which pleases me and my doctor to no end.

Before surgery for my staph infection, my hair was falling out, but since learning to eat right, my hair is coming back thicker and is a lot easier to take care of. I recommend this program to anyone.

### SHARON VON GUNTEN

In March 2003, I was rushed to the hospital because I couldn't catch my breath. Doctors diagnosed me with congestive heart failure and Type II diabetes. (Dad died at age forty-eight from congestive heart failure, and Mom had diabetes before her death at the age of sixty-six.) Back then, I prayed and asked the Lord what to do. That's when I changed my diet to one of whole natural foods: no more deep-fried meals, less salt, a lot less sugar, and nothing highly processed. I lost eighty pounds over the next three years.

Then I attended the 7 Weeks of Wellness classes because I wanted to fine-tune my diet and upgrade my health another notch. I lost another six pounds in seven weeks. After wearing a size XXXX for many years, I'm now between XX and an XL, depending on the style of garment and where I buy my clothes. I also stopped taking all of my medications for diabetes and congestive heart disease because my cardiac specialist said my heart was no longer enlarged and beats perfectly now.

Best of all, I can sleep all the way through the night. For ten years, I would try to sleep in my own bed, but after dozing for an hour or so, I'd wake up and go sit in my recliner, where I could fall asleep again. After finishing the program, I started sleeping all the way through—in my own bed! I don't hear anything, and now I wake up when the alarm clock says it's time to get up.

### BEV HARRIS

I've had a thyroid disorder for twenty years, which has given me very dry skin. When the weather turns cold, my elbows and knuckles would crack and bleed if I didn't keep lotion on them. My scalp has been itchy too.

Since I began following the Great Physician's Rx and eating organic foods, cooking with coconut oil, and supplying my body with organic fresh fruits, berries, avocados, and wild fish, my skin has a beautiful oil shine, and my hair actually has oil in it. Amazing! Better yet, I never knew food could taste so good, including fish, which I *never* used to eat.

I lost around five pounds—and two dress sizes—during the 7 Weeks of Wellness while eating more food than I ever have. I'm forty-eight years old but feel like I'm thirty again! Three months ago, I wasn't sleeping through the night because of night sweats and hot flashes, but now I can sleep almost every night all the way through and rarely have a hot flash.

I'm cooking at home, which my family loves, because they say the food is so delicious. I know that we will never go back to our old eating lifestyle because our new way of eating is too good, and, of course, it's good for my entire family.

### Bobbie Pezzoni

After hearing Jordan's teaching, I began implementing changes little by little, but eliminating artificial sweeteners was a big deal for me. I didn't realize how my "safe" choice of sweetener was affecting me until I quit using it. My sinuses cleared, and a couple of days later my migraine headaches ceased. At about week five into the program, my energy really increased, and my clothes felt looser. I can assure you that my desire for my old favorite foods dropped off as my taste buds changed, and I felt vitality for the first time in years.

### Caryn Edens

I haven't been able to work since 1993 because of vertigo and high blood pressure. Doctors have told me that I am a diabetic with fibromyalgia. I've had a cardiac catheterization, two upper endoscopies with biopsies, a colonoscopy, a retrograde pancreatography, pulmonary embolism, hysterectomy, both carpal tunnel releases, sinus surgery, and many MRIs over the years. When doctors found a tumor on of my adrenal glands, I was told that I had a one-in-six chance of dying during surgery to remove it. I agreed to undergo the procedure because it felt like I was dying from pain, but my long-term survival chances would be grim since I have only one adrenal gland remaining.

Since that surgery, I have been on pain medications and been housebound for years, with varying symptoms of pain and a low immune system.

Then I followed the 7 Weeks of Wellness program and saw major changes in my health, including the loss of twenty-five pounds. My mind became focused after hearing how to eat and live according to God's Word. I was taught that processed foods were empty of nutrition. I can assure you that I noticed a big reduction in my pain and swelling of face, hands, and feet when I started getting nutrition directly from the sources God Himself has provided. This program, with all of its helpful information, was just the piece of the puzzle that was missing from my life. Junk foods *really cost me* my health for a long time. I've noticed that people don't complain about the cost of chips and desserts, so why should they complain about the cost of life-giving foods?

I'll never forget trying omega-3 cod-liver oil for the first time. My girlfriend and I stood at the sink and filled a teaspoon and dared each other to try it . . . one . . . two . . . three . . . Go! We felt so brave, and it wasn't that bad. Her children were quick to grab a spoon and follow us.

The omega-3 cod-liver oil was not fishy, and it didn't upset my stomach, but I have to tell you what happened after taking omega-3 cod-liver oil. I wear glasses all the time; without them, I see very poorly. I even wore them when I took a shower. When I'd go to bed, I'd turn out the light and hear my husband's caring voice reminding me to take off my glasses.

After five days of taking a half teaspoon of omega-3 cod-liver oil, I could see without my glasses. I could read words on the television, which was amazing to me. But the best part hasn't been the improved eyesight, the increase in energy, or the loss in weight; it's been the reflection of Christ that rests on my life in a new way. Thank you, God, for answering the cry of my heart.

## CRISTI MURRAY

Ever since I was in a car accident in the summer of 1994, I've been struggling with chronic pain, depression, chronic fatigue, irritable bowel syndrome, sleep apnea, depression, fibromyalgia, and a sleep disorder. I got so discouraged and thought, *Lord, is this what the rest of my life will be like?* I could never lose weight with all the medications I had to take.

When Jordan Rubin spoke to us about the Great Physician's Rx, though, I could see with my own eyes how healthy he looked. Hope came alive for me. I thought, *What do I have to lose? Could this be what I have been praying for?*

I thought my husband, Kim, and I had been eating and living healthy until I started the 7 Weeks of Wellness classes. They were an eye-opener! Kim agreed to go along with the program, eating the healthy foods I prepared.

Midway through the health classes, I was really talking to the Lord about my irritable bowel syndrome, which has been a problematic discomfort for eleven years. I took medicine four times a day to deal with it. While in prayer one day, I felt the Lord was healing me of this affliction. I didn't tell anyone, but I continued to thank the Lord, in faith, that my healing would mean not taking any more medicine. From that day on, I've had no symptoms! Now I feel more free and confident in public places, and I'm motivated to continue my journey toward health and wellness.

I lost twenty pounds during the seven-week program, raised my energy level, and lowered my pain. I seem to be sleeping better at night, not waking up several times in the early morning with pain. The Great Physician's Rx has given me hope to achieve a healthier future—it is like a frame around a picture of good health. Now I'm looking forward to living life abundantly.

## HEATHER MCNICHOLS

I'm twenty-five years old and have been battling IBS and acid reflux since I was twelve. No amount of antacids or high-fiber diet could help. When I heard about the 7 Weeks of Wellness program, I decided to just go for it no matter how weird or crazy it sounded. Needless to say, my acid reflux, indigestion, and IBS have all subsided, and the only time they rear their ugly heads is when I eat something I shouldn't.

God is funny like that! I just turn to Him and say, *I know, I know,* and I get right back on track. I lost five pounds without trying during the seven weeks, but the best improvement has been my skin. I've had acne issues since I was a teen, but my skin has cleared up as well.

You know, I never used to make it through a day without a soda. Seriously! Today I'm soda-free and feel better than ever. I can also definitely tell the difference when I go to sleep before midnight and after midnight—a night-and-day difference. I just want to give God all the glory and praise and completely surrender my life to Him in *all* aspects.

### ASHLEY KNAPPER

I had been looking for a way to get healthier for a while. I knew that eating healthy and exercising was very important, but I needed some guidance. Jordan's message of the Great Physician's Rx was so inspirational and motivating that my mom and I decided to enroll in the 7 Weeks of Wellness program, where I learned how many foods that I ate every day were unhealthy. They seemed to be all the foods on the store shelf!

As I learned what foods would help me feel and be healthy, I began incorporating all seven keys from the Great Physician's Rx. I lost five pounds during the program and felt motivated to push on and keep strong with this program. Since taking the whole food multivitamins, omega-3 cod-liver oil, and green food, I can tell my body is running better. The advanced hygiene program has helped clear up my skin, which is very important for someone my age—nineteen. I have reduced my seasonal allergies as well.

I want to thank Jordan Rubin for his book and his guidance; it was just the help I needed to get back on the right foot of a healthy lifestyle.

### CAROL ANN RANGEL

Before the 7 Weeks of Wellness program, I was taking twelve to fourteen fiber capsules a day just to feel relief. Now that only good food is going into my body, I can miss two or three days of the fiber capsules before taking only two!

Most important, with this decision to change, my appetite for God has improved. I give God all the glory, honor, and praise now that I can serve Him with my mind, body, and soul.

### PATRICIA BOYD

I'm sixty-six years of age and do not have any major health problems—no diabetes, no cholesterol, for which I praise God. But when I heard Jordan Rubin and learned about the 7 Weeks of Wellness program, I jumped right in. The program has made me very aware of my diet, exercise, advanced hygiene, deep breathing, and most of all, my prayer life and my purpose in life.

I started going to the gym at our church twice a day, morning and afternoon, where I did functional fitness exercises that sent endorphins to my brain. In addition, I lost weight and inches around my midsection, which helped my overall physical well-being. I know that God does not make mistakes. He wants us to prosper and be in good health.

### MICHELE JURI

My children, who are now twelve, eleven, and nine years of age, were diagnosed with learning disabilities right around first and second grades. My pediatrician suggested I put my kids on Ritalin, but I had a feeling—call it mother's intuition—that I shouldn't do it.

Since then, I've tried many different vitamins and minerals, studied the psychology book about ADHD and different learning styles, but I have always struggled with my decision not to put my kids on a drug.

Long story short, I've had a few arguments with doctors over this one, but I knew I was doing the right thing. When the kids and I followed the 7 Weeks of Wellness program, I threw out all the unhealthy foods in my pantry and fridge and bought foods that God created. I noticed an immediate difference in each of the children—and so did their teachers. They said the boys were calmer, more focused in the classroom, and more at peace. Thank you, thank you!

Just so you know, I have ADD and started taking Adderall XR six months ago. Since changing my diet, under my doctor's care, I've been able to take my pills only two days a week instead of all seven. Yeah!

### Cindy Lunt

Ten years ago, my gastroenterologist told me I was lactose intolerant and had a digestive problem. I was put on a special diet called "restricted fiber and residue." This meant I was not allowed raw vegetables or fruits, berries, avocados, and whole-grain breads. I could only eat beef, chicken, bland white bread, and certain fruits if they were cooked.

Then I had gall bladder attacks, which resulted in the removal of my gall bladder last year and a reminder from my doctor: "No high-fat food."

When I heard about the Great Physician's prescription for health and wellness from Jordan Rubin, I made major changes over the next fifty days. I stopped drinking four Pepsis a day. I lost weight. I ate healthy, and better yet, I threw away that crazy food list my doctors gave me. My food digests properly now. I can eat berries, nuts, and wheat bread without getting sick. I was able to stop taking digestive meds. Thank you, Jordan, for writing your books and creating an awesome 7 Weeks of Wellness program. I feel so much better, and my body is functioning like a normal person's for the first time in my life, praise God!

### Alicia Hammond

From the age of thirteen, I've struggled with my fluctuating weight. I tried diet shakes, but they worked only as long as I was drinking them. Since I started the 7 Weeks of Wellness program, though, I've lost seven pounds, and the fat seems to be melting off of me. I know I've gained muscle, and my energy level is through the roof. The omega-3 cod-liver oil seems to be helping my metabolism, which is helping me physically and spiritually to be a better person.

### NICHOLL FRANCO

I have had a problem with regular bowel movements since I was in elementary school. In the last twenty years, I've tried natural fiber, holistic alternatives, fiber pills, colon cleanses, and finally, over-the-counter laxatives, which I have taken for the last ten years.

Since beginning the 7 Weeks of Wellness program, I've stopped taking laxatives and started becoming "regular." This has sincerely been a miracle and an answer to prayer. I know I will continue eating and living God's way.

### KIM MOSS

I'm not sure what drew me to go on the 7 Weeks of Wellness program. I'm forty-five years old, don't have allergies, haven't had the flu in over twenty years, and I seldom get a cold. I'm not overweight, and the only health problem I have is high cholesterol, which I'm managing with healthy diet and exercise. Or at least I thought I was eating a healthy diet before I began this program. I didn't know that opening up a jar of canned fruit or canned vegetables was a waste of time, or that margarine and processed foods were so unhealthy.

One day, I wanted to go to a Jamba Juice for a healthy fruit smoothie, but to save time, I stopped by a coffee place and ordered a strawberry smoothie because I wanted something "healthy." I watched the person behind the counter make my smoothie with nothing but artificial ingredients—one of the Dirty Dozen—and I didn't even get a single real strawberry. Two months ago I would have walked out of that coffee shop thinking I was drinking something healthy, but not now.

I'm doing my best to stay away from the Dirty Dozen and processed foods, which is my goal. Oh, and I did lose five pounds during the program, which is nothing to sneeze at.

## MAGGIE VENEZIO

During these seven weeks of the wellness program, I have been conscious of what goes into my mouth for the first time in my life. I no longer eat bacon, sausage, pork chops, crab, or lobster. And I'm working on avoiding the rest of the Dirty Dozen. I love water even more now, and now I only drink spring water, black tea, and kefir. I *love* kefir.

I truly enjoyed the 7 Weeks of Wellness, and I plan to continue eating to live.

## WENDI SMITH

I had gastric bypass surgery last year, and the vitamins the doctor recommended were horrible. I've really noticed a difference with the whole food multivitamins and with eating organic foods as recommended in the Great Physician's Rx.

## TERESA GUILLETTE

When I started the 7 Weeks of Wellness program, I was doubtful that the program could help me. Boy, was I wrong! I weighed 221 pounds when I started and weighed 202 pounds seven weeks later. I feel so much better. (So does my husband.)

Jordan's principles have changed my way of eating and living. I'm very conscious about eating healthy, God's way, but my favorite key is Key #7, "Living a Life of Prayer and Purpose." I thank the Lord for the opportunity to learn how to be healthier so He can use me for His will.

## JOLENE EMERSON

I've been married for ten years and am the mother of two children, a six-year-old boy and a four-year-old daughter.

When I heard about Jordan Rubin and the Great Physician's Rx, I was ready for a change because I was getting really overweight from really bad eating habits. I had been putting bad things in my body, and none of my clothes were fitting any longer. I was tired all the time and didn't have any energy. I think when you have kids that you have less time for yourself and let yourself go a little bit. That's what happened to me after I started my family.

I was ready for a change because I've struggled with my weight all my life. I was known as a cute, chubby little girl, but it's not so cute when you're twenty-eight years old. Being overweight depressed me, made me grumpy and crabby.

I tried lots of different fad diets, like the low-carb regimes that have been popular in recent years. I'd lose weight and then put it right back on—plus twenty more pounds. I think the reason why low-carb diets didn't work is because the minute I was done, I'd go back to eating the same thing as before and gain all that weight back. The hardest thing for me was sticking with something and following through with it.

Then I heard about The Great Physician's Rx. I was scared to adopt the Seven Keys because I'm the worst when it comes to eating bad things, but this time around I prayed before I started because I was filled with self-doubt and thoughts like, *You can't do this.*

I should have relaxed. Changing over from processed foods to a diet loaded with healthy meats, dairy, fruits, vegetables, and even desserts was easy—a lot easier than I thought it would be. After just one week, I had so much more energy. I felt good about myself because I was putting the right things into my body, not junk food that dragged down my energy levels.

Over the next couple of months of following the Great Physician's Rx, I lost twenty-two pounds, which was pretty awesome. I had to go shopping for clothes in smaller sizes, which was exciting. But my children, even at their young ages, could see a difference in me, which was really exciting.

Hopefully, they won't have to reach the age of twenty-eight before they learn the importance of good health.

*Jolene Emerson does not attend Calvary Temple Church because she and her family live in Carson, Washington.*

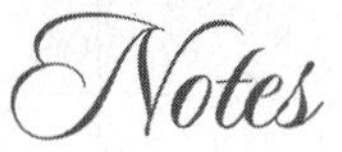

# Notes

## Introduction

1. "USA Statistics in Brief 2006," U.S. Census Bureau, available at http://www.census.gov/statab/www/brief.html.
2. "Biology Shows Women and Men Are Different," a press release issued by the Mayo Clinic in Scottsdale, Phoenix, on September 26, 2002, and available at http://www.mayoclinic.org/news2002-sct/1453.html.
3. James Dobson, *Love for a Lifetime* (Portland: Multnomah Press, 1987), 42–43, and based on research done by Dr. Paul Popenoe in his article, "Are Women Really Different?"
4. "Life Expectancy Hits Record High," a press release by the Centers for Disease Control Center for Health Statistics Press Office, issued February 28, 2005, and available at http://www.cdc.gov/nchs/pressroom/05facts/lifeexpectancy.htm.
5. Lawrence K. Altman, MD, "Is the Longer Life the Healthier One?" *New York Times*, Women's Health section, June 22, 1997, and available at http://www.nytimes.com/specials/women/nyt97/22altm.html.
6. "Women and Cardiovascular Disease: Mortality Trends for Males and Females," a statistical fact sheet compiled by the American Heart Association.
7. "Women's Top Health Threats: A Surprising List," http://www.mayoclinic.com/health/womens health/WO00014.
8. "The Heart Truth for Women," a press release issued by the National Heart, Lung, and Blood Institute, part of the National Institutes of Health. "The Heart Truth" is a national awareness campaign for women about heart disease and can be viewed online at http://www.nhlbi.nih.gov/health/hearttruth/.
9. American Cancer Society, *Cancer Facts and Figures 2005* (Atlanta: American Cancer Society, 2005).
10. Committee on Diet, Nutrition, and Cancer, Assembly of Life Sciences, National Research Council, Diet, Nutrition, and Cancer (Washington, D.C.: National Academy Press, 1982).
11. "Women's Top Health Threats," http://www.mayoclinic.com/health/womens-health/WO00014.
12. From the article, "Total Prevalence of Diabetes and Pre-Diabetes," found on the American Diabetes Association Web site at http://www.diabetes.org/diabetes-statistics/prevalence.jsp.
13. William R. Mattox Jr., "Nag, Nag, Nag: Does a Wife's Nagging Do a Man Good?" *Focus on the Family* magazine, April 1996, 10–11.

14. "Women More Proactive in Managing Their Health," a study performed by ACNielsen Canada, released November 13, 2003, at http://www.acnielsen.ca/News/Healthcare2003_WomenareMoreProactive.htm (site now discontinued).
15. "Women Are Catching Up to Men in Most Measures of Online Life," Pew/Internet press release issued December 28, 2005, and available at http://www.pewinternet.org/press_release.asp?r=119.

## KEY #1: EAT TO LIVE

1. "When It Pays to Buy Organic," *Consumer Reports*, February 2006, 12–15.
2. Marcus Kabel, Associated Press, "Wal-Mart Plans to Sell More Organic Merchandise," March 25, 2006.
3. Leah Hoffmann and Lacey Rose, "Costly Calories," *Forbes*, March 6, 2005, and available online at http://www.forbes.com/health/2005/04/06/cx_lrlh_0406costlycalories.html?boxes=custom.
4. "Organic Food Is More Nutritious Than Conventional Food," *Journal of Applied Nutrition*, 1993, 45:35–39, and available at http://www.organicconsumers.org/Organic/organicstudy.cfm.
5. Pat Volchok, "Going the Organic Way," *The Costco Connection* magazine, January 2006, 82.
6. Harvard School of Public Health, "Protein: Moving Closer to Center Stage," available at http://www.hsph.harvard.edu/nutritionsource/protein.html.
7. Jerry W. Thomas, "Restaurant Industry Losing the Low-Fat War," white paper from Decision Analyst, Inc., and available at http://www.decisionanalyst.com/publ_art/lowfat.asp.
8. Sally Fallon with Mary G. Enig, PhD, *Nourishing Traditions: The Cookbook That Challenges Politically Correct Nutrition and the Diet Dictocrats* (Washington, D.C.: NewTrends Publishing, 2000), www.newtrendspublishing.com.
9. "Kraft Slashes Trans Fat in Time for Labeling Deadline," from Food & Drink Europe.Com, issued online on December 23, 2005.
10. Arne Astrup, Thomas Meinert Larsen, and Angela Harper, SkepticReport.com, "Atkins and Other Low-Carbohydrate Diets," available at http://www.skepticreport.com/health/atkins.htm.
11. Nichola Groom, Reuters News Service, "Atkins Files for Bankruptcy as Low-Carb Slumps," August 1, 2005.
12. Karen Pallaritio, "Iron Pills May Boost Brain Function in Women," *HealthDay*, April 19, 2004, found at http://www.hon.ch.
13. Jean Carper, "Mighty Magnesium," *USA Today Weekend*, September 1, 2002, and available at http://www.usaweekend.com/02_issues/020901/020901eatsmart.html.
14. Ibid.
15. Tori Hudson, ND, *Women's Encyclopedia of Natural Medicine*, (Lincolnwood, IL: Keats, 1999), 184–85.
16. *The Encyclopedia of Natural Healing* (Burnaby, BC, Canada: Alive Publishing Group, Inc., 1997), 948.
17. *Vaginal Yeast Infections*, a booklet produced by the National Women's Health Information Center of the U.S. Department of Health and Human Services, and available at http://www.4woman.gov/faq/yeastinfect.htm.
18. F. Batmanghelidj, MD, *You're Not Sick, You're Thirsty!* (New York: Warner Books, 2003), 225–26.

19. H. J. Roberts, *The Aspartame Problem,* statement for Committee on Labor and Human Resources, U.S. Senate hearing on NutraSweet—Health and Safety Concerns, November 3, 1987, 83–178 (Washington, DC: U.S. Government Printing office, 1988), 466–67.

20. Elizabeth Querna, "One Sweet Nation," *U.S. News & World Report,* March 28, 2005, http://www.usnews.com/usnews/health/articles/050328/28sugar.b.htm.

21. From the Daily Celebrations Web site for December 29, http://www.dailycelebrations.com/122999.htm.

22. "The Sum of Chocolate," a press release issued December 20, 2005, by FoodProductionDaily.com.

23. Rex Russell, *What the Bible Says About Healthy Living* (Ventura, CA: Regal, 1996), 154.

24. Paula Moore, "Hot Dog! Devoting a Month to a Disgusting Sack of Pork," *Philadelphia Inquirer,* July 10, 2001.

25. "Facts and Figures," a press release issued by the National Pork Producers Council and available at http://www.nppc.org/resources/facts.html.

26. Stephan Jack, "China: A Nation of Pork Eaters," http://www.eatingchina.com/articles/art-pork.html.

## KEY #2: SUPPLEMENT YOUR DIET WITH WHOLE FOOD NUTRITIONALS, LIVING NUTRIENTS, AND SUPERFOODS

1. *Encyclopedia of Natural Healing,* 194–95.

2. Phyllis A. Balch, CNC, *Prescription for Nutritional Healing* (Wayne, NJ: Avery Publishing: 2000), 2.

3. Gina Kolata, "Vitamins: More May Be Too Many," *New York Times,* April 29, 2004.

4. *Encyclopedia of Natural Healing,* 194–95.

5. Annette Dickinson, PhD, "*The Benefits of Nutritional Supplements,*" a report issued by the Council for Responsible Nutrition, July 2002.

6. Angela Fernandez, "Vitamania," *Image,* November 2005, 16.

7. James F. Balch, MD, and Mark Stengler, ND, *Prescription for Natural Cures* (Hoboken, NJ: John Wiley & Sons, Inc., 2004), 550.

8. Kathleen Fairfield, MD, and Robert Fletcher, MD, "Vitamins for Chronic Disease Prevention: Scientific Review and Clinical Applications," Clinician's Corner, *Journal of the American Medical Association,* 287, no. 23 (June 19, 2002).

9. Daniel H. Chong, ND, "Real or Synthetic: The Truth Behind Whole Food Supplements," http://www.mercola.com/2005/jan/19/whole_food_supplements.htm.

10. Ingrid B. Helland, MD, et al., "Maternal Supplementation with Very-Long-Chain n-3 Fatty Acids During Pregnancy and Lactation Augments Children's IQ at 4 Years of Age," *Pediatrics,* 111, no. 1 (January 2003), e39–e44.

11. M. S. LeBoff et al., "Occult Vitamin D Deficiency in Postmenopausal U.S. Women with Acute Hip Fracture," *Journal of the American Medical Association,* 251(1999), 1505–11.

12. Richard Hobday, *The Healing Sun* (Scotland, UK: Findhorn Press, 1999), 59–60.

13. Salynn Boyles, "Vitamin D May Lower Some Cancer Risk," *WebMD Medical News,* December 28, 2005, http://www.webmd.com/content/article/116/112304.htm.

14. William B. Grant, "Breast Cancer: Risk and Risk Reduction Factors," http://www.sunarc.org/breastcan402.htm.
15. John R. Lee, MD, *What Your Doctor May Not Tell You About Menopause: The Breakthrough Book on Natural Progesterone* (New York: Warner Books, 1996), 9.
16. Star Lawrence, "Making the Most of Eating Green Food," http://www.webmd.com/content/article/101/106435.htm.
17. Ibid.
18. Michael T. Murray, ND, and Jade Beutler, RRT, *Fats and Oils: Your Guide to Healing with Essential Fatty Acids* (Ferndale, WA: Apple Publishing, 1996).
19. T. Norat, *Journal of the National Cancer Institute*, June 15, 2005, 906–16, news release, National Cancer Institute, http://my.webmd.com/content/article/107/108494.htm.
20. Dr. Johanna Budwig, *Flax Oil as a True Aid Against Arthritis, Heart Infarction, Cancer, and Other Diseases* (Canada: Apple Publishing, 1994).
21. "Flaxseed," American Cancer Society Web site, and available at http://www.cancer.org/docroot/ETO/content/ETO_5_3X_Flaxseed.asp?sitearea=ETO.
22. Carolyn Strange, "Boning Up on Osteoporosis," http://www.webmd.com/content/article/7/1680_51715.htm.
23. "Health News," published online by Harvard Medical School's Consumer Health Information Web site, http://www.intelihealth.com/IH/ihtIH/WSIHW000/333/8988/455014.html.
24. Colette Bouchez, "Looking Good—From the Inside Out," http://www.webmd.com/content/article/86/99208.htm.
25. Ibid.

## KEY #3: PRACTICE ADVANCED HYGIENE

1. S. Minz, "Childbirth in Early America," 2003, http://www.digitalhistory.uh.edu/historyonline/childbirth.cfm.
2. From a 2003 study sponsored by the American Society of Microbiology as part of its "Take Action: Clean Hands Campaign," http://www.asm.org/Media/index.asp?bid=21773.
3. Lisa Petrillo, "SDSU Study: Germs Hitch Ride in Plane Bathrooms," *San Diego Union-Tribune*, December 26, 2005.
4. C. J. McManus and S. T. Kelley, "Molecular Survey of Aeroplane Bacterial Contamination," *Journal of Applied Microbiology*, 99 (March 2005), 502–508, doi: 10.1111/ j.1365-2672.2005.02651.x.
5. "More People Fear Germs in Restrooms than Any Other Public Place," a survey conducted by Opinion Research Corporation International on behalf of Kimberly-Clark Professional and issued as a press release on October 17, 2001.
6. "Germ Survey: Summary of Findings," conducted in May 2004 by Opinion Research Corporation and available at uanews.org/pdfs/germsurvey.
7. "Flu Season Is Here," a press release issued by PR Newswire Association, October 6, 2005, and available at http://www.keepmedia.com/pubs/PRNewswire/2005/10/06/1039338.
8. "Ewww! Don't Touch That Mouse!" *The Age*, February 15, 2006, and available at http://www.theage.com.au/articles/2006/02/15/1139890812017.html.

9. Kenneth Seaton, PhD, "A New Way to Prevent Colds and Flu," *Health Freedom News*, March 1992, 14.
10. From the Medical Institute's "Frequently Asked Questions" Web page, which is available at http://www.medinstitute.org/health/questions_answers.html.
11. Tim and Beverly LaHaye, *The Act of Marriage After 40* (Grand Rapids: Zondervan, 2000).
12. Paul Farhi, "In Flu Season, the Handshake Loses Favor," *Washington Post*, December 25, 2004.
13. Ibid.

## KEY #4: CONDITION YOUR BODY WITH EXERCISE AND BODY THERAPIES

1. National Sleep Foundation, "Women's Unique Sleep Experiences," http://www.sleepfoundation.org/hottopics/index.php?secid=17&id=163.
2. From the National Sleep Foundation Web site and the article, "Can't Sleep? Learn About Insomnia," which is available at http://www.sleepfoundation.org/sleeplibrary/index.php?secid=&id=58.
3. The National Heart, Lung, and Blood Institute, "Insomnia," publication no. 95–3801, October 1995.
4. Colorado Neurological Institute, "New Sleep Medicines and Treatments," http://www.thecni.org/s-sleep_disorders.htm.
5. Stephanie Saul, "Surge in Ads Drives Sales of the Latest Sleep Pills," *New York Times*, February 7, 2006.
6. Balch, *Prescription for Nutritional Healing*, 474.
7. Christen Brownlee, "Buff and Brainy: Exercising the Body Can Benefit the Mind," *Science News* magazine, February 25, 2006, and available at http://www.sciencenews.org/articles/20060225/bob10.asp.
8. J. Bartholomew, *Medicine & Science in Sports & Exercise*, 2005; vol 37: 2032–37. University of Texas at Austin, with commentary by Jennifer Warner of WebMD Medical News, news release, "Exercise May Lift Cloud of Depression, http://www.webmd.com/content/article/117/112688?printing=true.
9. Jeannine Stein, "The Amish Paradox," *Los Angeles Times*, January 12, 2004.
10. Charles Stuart Platkin, "Counting Steps with Pedometer Seems to Encourage Fitness," *Honolulu Advertiser*, March 24, 2004.
11. Betsy McCormack, *Fit Over 40 for Dummies* (Foster City, CA: IDG Books, 2001), 54.
12. Tim Layden, "I Am an American," *Sports Illustrated*, October 31, 2005, 61–62.
13. "Happy Birthday, Mr. President," from the *Cavalier Daily*, available at http://www.cavalierdaily.com/CVArticle.asp?ID=19730&pid=1150.
14. Douglas Duper and Teresa Odle, "Essential Oils," *The Gale Encyclopedia of Alternative Medicine*, October 25, 2005, and available at http://www.keepmedia.com/pubs/EncyclopediaOfAlternativeMedicine/2005/10/25/1142454?ba=a&bi=0&bp=7.
15. Ibid.
16. Joan Raymond and Jerry Adler, "A Neglected Nutrient: Are Americans Dying from a Lack of Vitamin D?" *Newsweek*, January 17, 2005.

17. Alex Raksin, "Making a Case for Sun's Benefits," *Los Angeles Times*, June 20, 2005.
18. Marilynn Marchione, "Scientists Say Sunshine May Prevent Cancer," Associated Press, May 21, 2005 (article no longer available on site).
19. "Tanning Booths: Are They Worth the Risk?" http://womenshealth.about.com/od/dermatology/l/aa04219.htm.

## KEY #5: REDUCE TOXINS IN YOUR ENVIRONMENT

1. Douglas Fischer, "What's in You?" *Oakland Tribune*, March 18, 2005, and available at http://www.insidebayarea.com/bodyburden/ci_2600879.
2. Ibid.
3. Centers for Disease Control and Prevention, *Third National Report on Human Exposure to Environmental Chemicals*, NCEH Pub. No. 05–0570.
4. "Companion Report to CDC's 2005 National Exposure Report," a press release issued by Physicians for Social Responsibility.
5. "What You Need to Know About Starting Bioidentical Hormone Therapy (BHRT)," found on the official Web site of John R. Lee, MD, at http://www.johnleemd.com/store/get_off_hrt.html.
6. Liz Lipski, PhD, CCN, "Basics of Nutrition and Healthy Eating," http://www.womentowomen.com/nutritionandweightloss/nutritionalbasics.asp.
7. "Are Artificial Sweeteners Safe?" http://www.webmd.com/content/Article/102/106833.htm?pagenumber=5.
8. Kelly James-Enger, "Sweet Stuff: How Artificial Sweeteners May Affect Your Stomach," http://acidreflux.msn.com/article.aspx?aid=64>1=7338 (site now discontinued).
9. Justin Gillis, "Bionic Growth for Biotech Crops," *Washington Post*, January 12, 2006, D1.
10. "Americans' Knowledge of Genetically Modified Foods Remains Low," a press release issued by Pew Research, November 15, 2005, and available at http://www.pewtrusts.org/ideas/ideas_item.cfm?content_item_id=3123&content_type_id=7&page=7&issue=12&issue_name=Food%20&%20Biotechnology&name=Grantee%20Press%20Releases&source=yahoo&OVRAW=Genetically%20Modified%20Food&OVKEY=genetically%20modified%20food&OVMTC=standard.
11. Linda Bren, "Genetic Engineering: The Future of Foods?" *FDA Consumer*, November–December 2003, and available at http://www.fda.gov/fdac/features/2003/603_food.html.
12. "When It Pays to Buy Organic," *Consumer Reports*, February 2006, 12.
13. Jim Robbins, "Think Global, Eat Local," *Los Angeles Times Magazine*, July 31, 2005, 9–10.
14. David Steinman and Samuel S. Epstein, MD, *The Safe Shopper's Bible* (New York: Wiley Publishing, 1995), 18.
15. http://www.mercola.com/forms/air_purifiers.htm.
16. "Dust Mites: Common Cause of Allergy Symptoms," http://www.mayoclinic.com/health/dustmites/HQ00864, June 17, 2005.
17. Sandra Felton, the "Organization Lady," is founder of Messies Anonymous and author of many organizing books, including *The Messie Manual* and *Organizing Magic*. Her Web site is www.messies.com.

18. From a National Aeronautics and Space Administration study, "Interior Landscape Plants for Indoor Air Pollution Abatement," released September 15, 1989.
19. Mindy Pennybacker, "Healthier Home Cleaning," *The Green Guide*, September 8, 2003.
20. Ibid.
21. Ibid.
22. David Rubien, "The Sticking Point," *San Francisco Chronicle*, June 15, 2005.
23. Reg Ponniah, "Facts Won't Stick to Teflon," PlaNet News and Views Web site, available at http://www.pl.net/Nhealth/factel.htm.
24. Rubien, "The Sticking Point."
25. Juliet Eilperin, "Harmful Teflon Chemical to Be Eliminated by 2015," *Washington Post*, January 26, 2006, A1.
26. The *Wall Street Journal* report was a video found on www.mercola.com, and is available at http://www.mercola.com/forms/light_bulbs.htm#.
27. Plant Management in Florida Waters, "Freshwater Consumption in Florida," press release, available at http://aquat1.ifas.ufl.edu/guide/drinking.html.
28. Ibid.
29. Raina Kelly, "Return of a Silent Killer," *Newsweek*, February 21, 2005.
30. Steinman and Epstein, *The Safe Shopper's Bible*, 181.
31. Ibid.
32. Forbes.com, "Could Antiperspirants Raise Breast Cancer Risk?" http://www.forbes.com/lifestyle/health/feeds/hscout/2006/03/06/hscout531342.html, March 6, 2006.
33. Roger Vincent, "Organic Beauty Products Get a Lift with USDA About-Face," *Los Angeles Times*, August 25, 2006, C1.
34. Barry Meier, "Dow Chemical Deceived Women on Breast Implants, Jury Decides," *New York Times*, August 19, 1997.
35. Marc Kaufman, "Implant Maker Fixed Samples Only," *Washington Post*, December 5, 2005, A3, and available at http://www.washingtonpost.com/wp-dyn/content/article/2005/12/04/AR2005120400887.html?nav=rss_health.
36. "Shaping the Perfect Teenager," from the CBS TV show *48 Hours*, from the CBS Web site at http://www.cbsnews.com/stories/1999/05/25/48hours/main48474.shtml.
37. American Cancer Society, *Cancer Facts and Figures 2005* (Atlanta: American Cancer Society, 2005).
38. *Encyclopedia of Natural Healing*, 247.

## KEY #6: AVOID DEADLY EMOTIONS

1. Jane E. Brody, "Personal Health: Diagnosing PMS," *New York Times*, August 28, 1996.
2. Ellen W. Freeman, PhD, "Understanding PMS," an article on the University of Pennsylvania Health System Web site, http://www.vpul.upenn.edu/shs/
3. *Encyclopedia of Natural Healing*, 1067.
4. Hudson, *Women's Encyclopedia of Natural Medicine*, 250.
5. Phyllis A. Balch, *Prescription for Nutritional Healing*, 589.

6. "Let's Talk About Anxiety Disorders," a 2005 press release from the American Psychiatric Association, and available at http://www.healthyminds.org/multimedia/anxietydisorders.pdf.
7. Balch, *Prescription for Nutritional Healing,* 314–315.
8. Don Colbert, MD, *Deadly Emotions* (Nashville: Thomas Nelson, 2003), 63.
9. Ibid., 63–64.
10. Balch, *Prescription for Nutritional Healing,* 315.
11. "Panic Attack, Depression Harm Your Mind and Body," http://www.mercola.com/2005/oct/13/panic_attacks_depression_harm_your_mind_and_body.htm.
12. Shankar Vedantam and Marc Kaufman, "Doctors Influenced by Mention of Drug Ads," *Washington Post,* April 27, 2005, A1.
13. "Spousal Spats Can Damage Your Heart," Reuters News, March 3, 2006.
14. Ochsner Clinic Foundation news release, March 11, 2005, http://www.ochsner.org/HealthNews/Healthday.
15. "Panic Attack, Depression Harm Your Mind and Body," http://www.mercola.com/2005/oct/13/panic_attacks_depression_harm_your_mind_and_body.htm.
16. Patsy Clairmont, interview by Mike Yorkey, *Women of Faith* magazine, 2000.
17. Laurie Barclay, "'Baby Blues' Don't Have to Grow to Full-Blown Depression," http://www.webmd.com/content/article/31/1728_77400.htm.


## KEY #7: LIVE A LIFE OF PRAYER AND PURPOSE


1. "What Makes Prayer Work," from the National Day of Prayer Web site, http://www.ndptf.org/story/Index.cfm?Entity=9&Department=9&Dept_Order=1&This_Topic Order=13&This_SubtopicOrder=1.
2. Germaine Copeland, *Prayers That Avail Much* (Tulsa, OK: Harrison House, 1997) 228.
3. Beverly LaHaye, foreword to *The Christian Mom's Answer Book,* compiled and edited by Mike Yorkey and Sandra P. Aldrich (Colorado Springs, Colorado: Cook Communications, 1999), 15.

# About the Authors

**Jordan Rubin** has dedicated his life to transforming the health of others, one life at a time.

Jordan, thirty-one, is the founder and chairman of Garden of Life, Inc., a health-and-wellness company based in West Palm Beach, Florida, which produces organic foods, whole food nutritional supplements and personal care products.

He and his wife, Nicki, are the parents of their son, Joshua. They make their home in Palm Beach Gardens, Florida.

**Nicki Rubin** earned her MBA degree from Morehead State University in Morehead, Kentucky, before joining one of the Big 5 accounting firms, Arthur Andersen, as a certified public accountant. She left Arthur Andersen when she and Jordan started Garden of Life. Today Nicki is a stay-at-home mom and loving every minute of it.

**Pancheta Wilson, MD**, is a family and complementary medicine physician practicing in Coral Springs, Florida. She is a graduate of the West Indies Medical School, with postgraduate training in the Brooklyn and Meharry medical hospitals. Dr. Wilson is the author of several wellness books, including *Free Yourself from Diabetes.*

# Acknowledgments

Many others have played important roles in the *Great Physician's Rx for Women's Health*, including my wife, Nicki, who agreed to lend a hand to this massive project. Thank you, Nicki, for contributing so much time and effort to this book when you didn't have much time to give.

We were greatly aided by my writing partner and editor, Mike Yorkey, who's one of the best in the business. The more we write together, the more I think we're beginning to share the same brain.

I would like to thank the executive leadership at Thomas Nelson—Mike Hyatt, Jonathan Merck, and Ted Squires—who have made me feel a part of the Nelson family. Victor Oliver has also been a part of the editorial process from the early days. And I certainly appreciate the skill that Kristen Parrish, a Thomas Nelson editor, displayed in honing this manuscript.

Tina Jacobson and Kevin Small, my literary co-agents, continue to help me tremendously with their wisdom and experience.

And finally, I'd like to thank the Great Physician, my Lord and Savior Yeshua Ha Mashiach, Jesus the Messiah, who was and is and is to come. Any chance of success this book has rests entirely upon Him.